SMART FACE

ALSO BY THOMAS GOODMAN, M.D.:

The Skin Doctor's Skin Doctoring Book

SMART FACE

A DERMATOLOGIST'S GUIDE TO SAVING YOUR MONEY AND SAVING YOUR SKIN

Thomas Goodman, M.D.
and
Stephanie Young

PRENTICE HALL PRESS

NEW YORK LONDON TORONTO SYDNEY TOKYO

The information in this book is not intended to replace the services of a trained health professional or serve as a replacement for medical care. Consult your physician or health-care professional before following the author's proposed courses of treatment. The product listings in this book have been collected for the convenience of the reader and do not constitute a recommendation or endorsement of any product.

 Prentice Hall Press
Gulf + Western Building
One Gulf + Western Plaza
New York, New York 10023

Copyright © 1988 by Thomas Goodman, M.D. and Stephanie Young

PRENTICE HALL PRESS and colophon are registered
trademarks of Simon & Schuster, Inc.

Library of Congress Cataloging-in-Publication Data

Goodman, Thomas.

Smart face.

Includes index.
1. Skin—Care and hygiene.   2. Face—Care and
hygiene.   I. Young, Stephanie, 1956–   . II. Title.
RL87.G64   1988   616.5   88-6004
ISBN 0-13-814377-3

Designed by Stanley S. Drate/Folio Graphics Co., Inc.

Manufactured in the United States of America

10 9 8 7 6 5 4 3 2

ACKNOWLEDGMENTS

Persons who helped put this book together are sincerely thanked:

Stephanie Young, my coauthor, who transformed this work in a very short time from a too-medical and at times too-critical book into a complete consumer guide to the selection and use of cosmetics. Her skills as a writer and beauty expert are evident; they greatly broadened the dimensions of the book.

Susan Clark Companiotte, who served as valuable first reader. Her encouragement, her intelligence, and her understanding helped shape the form and direction of the book.

Barbara Lurie, Frances McPherson, and Mary Radford, who are this dermatologist's office staff and were involved with the production of the work.

Susan Powell, who typed most of the manuscript.

Madeline Collins, who produced the illustrations.

Faith Hornby of the Carol Mann Agency, our literary agent for this book.

—THOMAS GOODMAN, M.D.

My thanks to Thomas Goodman, M.D., coauthor, for his humor and patience, for understanding that detailed information on cosmetics is integral to a dermatologist's expertise, and above all for his welcoming a beauty writer's perspective.

—STEPHANIE YOUNG

CONTENTS

PART TWO

Skin Care

PART THREE

Skin Problems

INTRODUCTION

QUESTION:
> Can the new scientific breakthroughs in skin care really change my skin? Can collagen, cell renewal, overnight repair, cellular extracts, and concentrates reverse or prevent the signs of aging in my skin?

ANSWER:
> Almost surely not. There is little real evidence that these much-advertised "miracles" can do anything but temporarily improve the very thin surface layer of skin. Much of this book is devoted to showing you enough real facts about how skin and skin-care products work so that you will be smarter than the cosmetics makers and sellers seem to want you to be. The skin-care business contains a very large amount of hype. Small and insignificant "scientific" discoveries are taken and blown into major advertising campaigns.

Would you like your facial skin to be as beautiful and healthy as it can be? Are you tired of the unkept promises made by skin-care product advertisements? Would you like to feel you know enough about facial skin and its care so that *you*, and not the sellers of cosmetics and skin-care products, can make informed choices about the products your skin really needs?

This book is about caring for facial skin intelligently and well. It is about developing a real understanding of your facial skin and its problems. It is about how simple and inexpensive skin care can be as good as the very complex and sometimes exorbitantly expensive regimens that are usually recommended. And it is about helping you, the reader, develop a skin-care program that really suits your unique facial skin.

This book is written primarily for women, because they spend more time and money on facial skin care than men do. And, as any dermatologist would testify, women simply have more facial skin problems—often related to the normal hormonal changes through life, as well as to the use of skin-care products.

Even though women are the major consumers of cosmetic and skin-care products, they are at a disadvantage in the marketplace. So little has been done to help women really understand their facial skin that most are easy marks for the sellers of cosmetic and skin-care products. Modern skin-care products are so nicely packaged and so skillfully marketed, and advertising claims for them seem so "scientific," so "high tech," that women are easily influenced.

Makers of cosmetics and skin-care products, while producing beautiful and truly high-quality *products,* have gone beyond making legitimate promises on beautifying skin into a fantasy land of assurances that their new products can actually rebuild, restructure, and renew facial skin. You have read all the claims for cell renewal, reversing the aging process, firming, smoothing, and so on. Many of these claims are misleading or worse.

So this book is also about cosmetic and skin-care products, the claims made for them, and what can realistically be expected of them. Coupled with a better understanding of facial skin, that just might give you the feeling that you—and not the sellers of cosmetic and skin-care products—are actually in control of your own facial skin.

AN OVERVIEW OF THIS BOOK

Part I: "Understanding Facial Skin." Many people have almost no knowledge of the basic facts about skin. Misconceptions about the fundamentals are the rule rather than the exception. Considering the large amount of time, money, and pampering spent on facial skin, it is a sad truth. Start with chapter 1, "Facial Skin Through the Years, Seasons, and Days." Then read chapter 2, "Structure of the Skin," and the following chapters on wrinkles, pores, dry skin, and oily skin. Understanding these topics is absolutely essential if you want to be knowledgeable and sensible about facial skin care.

This section will help to open your eyes, clear up some misconceptions, and introduce objectivity and reality in analyzing your facial skin and evaluating cosmetic and skin-care product advertisements.

Part II: "Skin Care," discusses sun protection, cleansing, moisturizing, and foundation makeup. This will help you evaluate the confusing array of hundreds of products and make the whole issue of skin care easy to understand. You will learn what is good, useless, overpriced, and, most important, appropriate for *your* skin.

The manufacturers of skin-care and cosmetic products, and the people who advertise and sell them, have not been very helpful in educating the public about facial skin care. They are, after all, out to sell their products and that gets in the way of objectivity. The general public, and women in particular, are not getting good skin-care advice. What they *are* getting is thoroughly confused by misleading advertising claims. Things are becoming even more confusing with the attempts by the cosmetic companies to dazzle women with those scientific-sounding statements that seem to promise everything. The age of high tech is here—they are putting *computers* at cosmetic counters. How can anyone resist buying a product if a computer tells us it is needed?

Dermatologists, too, can be faulted in this regard. Masters at treating the ills of skin, most of them ignore the issues of skin care and cosmetics; they are somehow above it all. This attitude has allowed the cosmetic companies to take the lead in "educating" the public.

So learn about sensible skin care, and what skin-care products can do and cannot do. Spend no more money and time than you really want or need to, and still get excellent skin care.

Part III: "Skin Problems" is about all the common things that go wrong with facial skin. There is an extensive discussion of acne and breakout problems. This is a big problem for so many women twenty-five to forty-five years old. New information is given here about how hormones affect the acne problem.

Another chapter in this section worth special mention is chapter 15, "Seborrheic Dermatitis." This is a very prevalent facial problem that, it seems, is never understood by skin-care "experts" or by individuals who have it. It is a condition that occurs only on oily skin but is always thought to be a dry-skin problem.

And there are chapters on pigmentation problems, facial veins, perioral dermatitis, rosacea, eyelid dermatitis, and cosmetic reactions.

Especially now that there are more good nonprescription medications available to the public, really effective do-it-yourself home care is a reality. Instructions are given, where appropriate, about what medications to buy and how to use them. You should never delay in consulting a dermatologist if you need to, but there are many facial skin problems that are perfectly amenable to informed home treatment.

PART ONE

Understanding Facial Skin

FACIAL SKIN THROUGH THE YEARS, SEASONS, AND DAYS

1

QUESTION:
   What can I do to get great-looking skin and keep it that way?
ANSWER:
   There's no one right answer for this, because skin has changing needs through the years, seasons, and days. The key to
   having and maintaining better-looking skin is to be aware of
   when, how, and why your skin's needs change.

Facial skin is in a continuous state of change—day to day, month to month, season to season, year to year—evolving from the fresh, new, fine-textured skin of infancy into the sagging, wrinkling, weathered skin of old age. Smart skin care entails gaining some perspective about where your facial skin is now and where it may be going.

SKIN CHANGES THROUGH THE YEARS

Through the years, many of the same factors influence and affect the facial skins of all of us. Those major factors are hormone changes, sun exposure, and time. However, how such factors affect the look of our skins depends largely on inherited genetic traits.

Infancy to Teenage

These are usually the happiest years for facial skin. The new, clear, fine-textured skin of infancy and childhood is a thing of beauty. There are some little skin problems of infancy—those caused by the presence

3

of maternal hormones—but they are temporary and leave no permanent marks or scars.

Some children can develop acne problems before the teenage years, and it usually signals early pubertal hormone changes. Significant acne before the teen years should always be seen by a physician, as real hormonal abnormalities may be responsible.

The most significant factor affecting skin's future at this age is sunlight. Ultraviolet radiation damage starts as soon as sunlight strikes skin. Facial skin aging starts in childhood and can be prevented only by starting sun protection now. (More about this later, in chapter 8.)

Adolescence—Ages Thirteen to Seventeen

This is the first time for really dramatic skin changes. Just how dramatic and problematic depends upon the individual, but all facial skin does change in some way. All these major changes are due to the surge of sex hormones that occurs at this time. Both male and female hormones are produced in both boys and girls. While female hormones begin to change body shape and appearance, male hormones affect the oil glands of the face (as well as the back and chest).

Male hormones are the culprits in the skin changes and troubles of adolescence, as they cause the enlargement and increased activity of oil glands. Acne problems seem to come from the rapid enlargement of oil glands and increased oil production in immature skin. The very small pores of the child's skin just can't handle this rapid increase in oil. Blocked pores, blackheads, whiteheads, and pustules (all of these are included in what dermatologists call "acne") result.

Dandruff (seborrheic dermatitis of the scalp) and seborrheic dermatitis of the face, because they are problems of oily skin, may also develop during these years.

Young Adulthood—Ages Seventeen to Twenty-Seven

As the dramatic changes of adolescene are completed, as pores become larger and oil gland size and function stabilize, most of the adolescent skin woes cease. Some individuals aren't so lucky—they continue to have acne problems past adolescence. The skin just never seems to adjust itself to the higher oil-production levels. Such individuals are genetically disposed to produce lots of oil, or to have fine-textured skin with pores that just won't seem to enlarge enough to accommodate the increased oil flow.

Still, this is a time of more changes in the facial skin of females, due to hormone alterations. This is the time when women may be taking birth-control pills and be affected by the major hormone shifts associated with their use. And it is the time of pregnancy and the shifting hormone levels before, during, and after giving birth. Those hormone shifts change oil gland function and may produce more problems with acne breakouts.

This is the time when sun damage may begin to show up (especially for pale skin types), in the form of dilated ("broken") veins or capillaries around the nose or on the cheeks, superficial fine-line crinkling, and lentigines—splotches of pigment change easily mistaken for freckles.

Adulthood—Ages Twenty-Seven to Forty

This is the time of prime misunderstanding of facial skin. It is when accumulated sun exposure definitely begins to show up as lines and wrinkles. It is the time when many women apparently undergo another natural hormone shift, which results in a very unpleasant surprise—another period of acne breakouts. This is the time of maximum skin-care and cosmetic consciousness and expenditure. Ironically, it is also the time of much misunderstanding about appropriate skin care.

In spite of the development of lines and wrinkles, as many as half the women in this age group are developing skin that's oilier, not drier. The reemergence of breakout problems (statistics show that half of all females visiting dermatologists for acne are in this age group) and enlargement of pores are evidence of increasingly oily skin.

But it seems that all the cosmetic advertising is saying in boldface type and with endless repetition that skin at this age is drying out and needs *moisture*. Women rush to moisturize in the hopes of creaming away wrinkles. Unfortunately, "moisture" in cosmetics and skin-care products often means greasy substances that, when used on skins that are becoming more oily naturally, cause even more breakout problems. There is a thorough discussion of this in chapter 11.

Maturity—Ages Forty to Fifty

This is the decade in which wrinkles, lines, dilated surface veins and capillaries, skin cancers, precancers, and other benign growths come to the fore. It is the time when fair-skinned, light-eyed individuals are wishing they had been born with darker skin or had been more careful about sun exposure. It is the time of consulting dermatologists and plastic surgeons about collagen implants, face lifts, eyelid surgery, and the removal of various skin growths.

It is also a time of maximum gullibility about skin care. Those very expensive cosmetic and skin-care products that claim to "reverse the aging process" have an irresistible appeal as the signs of aging become more obvious.

Fifty Years and Beyond

During menopause and beyond, skin, like any other organ of the body, slows down some. The rate of repair and renewal of skin decelerates and decreases. The skin's top layer (stratum corneum) is significantly losing its moisture-holding ability. Oil gland activity is slowing down. Plumpness, strength, and resiliency of the deeper part of the skin (the dermis) diminishes. The result is a real increase in surface dryness (perhaps for the first time in a woman's life), as well as in wrinkling and sagging of the facial skin.

These changes stem from the natural aging process, a decline in female hormone levels, and from sun exposure.

Rosacea (an acnelike eruption of the face discussed more extensively in chapter 21) is a fairly rare problem in the population but most commonly develops in this age group. This condition is chronic and warrants special skin-care and cosmetic precautions. Rosacea can be, in some cases, directly related to the rapid hormonal declines at menopause. Whiteheads (tiny cysts deep in the skin) are another problem often seen in this age group.

And, of course, the benign and malignant skin growths continue to be a problem as years of sun exposure begin to surface. Actinic keratoses, seborrheic keratoses, basal and squamous skin cancers, lentigines, and dilated surface veins keep dermatologists busy.

Through trouble-free and troublesome stages, the evolution of skin through the years is a process we can only partially control. Not much can be done about time and genetics, but hormone changes can be partially modified and sun exposure resulting in skin damage can be controlled. It is for this reason that it is so important to get smart about using sunscreen products and limiting your time spent in the sun. How do skin care and cosmetics fit into the picture? Not as "magic potions" that can significantly change this evolution, but as the means to keep your skin fresh and healthy at any stage of life.

YOUR SKIN'S SEASONAL SHIFTS

Depending on your climate and your basic skin type, your skin can change dramatically—or less so—with the seasons.

Winter means drier skin for most people, due to colder temperatures, dry winds, and dry indoor heat. Oily types are least affected by these climatic changes, because the oil on the surface of the skin acts as a barrier to these drying influences. However, dry types can get very dry, sensitive types can get dry and irritated, and even normal types can become rougher and drier in texture.

In winter, always remember to protect your skin from the sun. Just because it's cold doesn't mean the sun's ultraviolet radiation isn't present—it is. Protection is especially important on the ski slopes—snow reflects radiation onto the face, and at higher elevations the atmosphere is thinner, so more radiation penetrates to the Earth's surface. Be cautious on vacation, too. While you may tote sun protection on your tropical getaway, be aware that the sun's rays get more intense the closer to the equator you go. It's a good idea to take an extra-high-SPF (sun-protection factor) sunscreen, as well as an alarm clock to time exposures on the beach and remind you when to reapply. Tropical breezes can keep you feeling cool while your skin is getting cooked.

Spring is a calm oasis for skin—winter's harshness is a fading memory and summer's heat is still in the future. All skin types can enjoy a few trouble-free months. Don't get lulled by the season's mildness—sunlight (and UV radiation) is getting stronger and lasting longer as days lengthen into summer.

Summer's warm sunny days signal the annual peaking of solar radiation reaching the earth, both in amount and in intensity. Appropriate skin-protection measures should be taken by everyone, from the very young to the more mature, from the very oily to the very dry.

One confusing side effect of summer's heat: The increase of perspiration, when it mingles with natural skin oils, leads some people to believe their skin is oilier. The fact is that oil and water don't mix, and oil floats to the top of the perspiration, producing an oilier look and feel to skin.

Another summer bugaboo is acne flare-up, caused by sun exposure. Ironically, some acne sufferers get better in the summer, experiencing fewer acne outbreaks. Ultraviolet radiation somehow makes the inflammation of acne less intense. However, for an unlucky few acne worsens after time in the sun. It is theorized that ultraviolet radiation and heat from the sun (or from a sunlamp or tanning booth) produce swelling of the skin around the sebaceous ducts, blocking them. Oil cannot flow freely to the skin surface, which encourages waxy plugs to form in the pores and acne to flare.

Fall is another season that's easy on most skin types, except for the acne-prone. Many experience a mid-September breakout, and it is theorized that this is a rebound reaction to excess sun exposure in summer. In general, this time of year is kind to most skin. Now's the season to practice some preventive skin care.

THE MONTHLY CYCLE OF SKIN CHANGES

Every twenty-eight days, your skin renews itself. That's how long it takes for new cells, produced in the basal layer, to migrate up and become the top layer of skin. As these skin cells move upward, they become smaller and flatter and eventually lifeless and form the outermost layer, the stratum corneum. They are then sloughed off.

For an average of three decades, the monthly ebb and flow of hormones affects the facial skin of women, some more than others. Anything from an isolated bump to a full-blown breakout can be the herald of menstruation. And if postperiod breakouts are more your pattern than preperiod ones, your skin disturbances signal the onset of ovulation. In short, any change in the balance of hormones can step up oil gland production and increase the likelihood of acne. This hormonally linked acne seems to disregard skin type; even normal skin can be troubled. Birth-control pills can sometimes tip the hormonal balance toward breakouts—and changing to a different one can also help prevent breakouts. (More about this in chapter 14.)

As you can see from this schedule of skin changes, there are plenty of ways to intervene in the look and health of your skin. It's the little, not necessarily expensive steps—like using sunscreens or washing when your skin needs it—that can mean great-looking skin for a lifetime. That's smart skin care.

STRUCTURE OF THE SKIN
Learning About the Layers

QUESTION:
How many layers are in my skin?
ANSWER:
You can get all sorts of answers to this question. We will keep it simple and say that there are three layers—stratum corneum, epidermis, and dermis. For purposes of understanding skin and its care, that is all you need to know. Some cosmetic advertising claims "penetration to the deepest layer." What they do *not* say is that they are talking about the deepest layer of the paper-thin top layer of skin.

Now for a short lesson in anatomy. The ten minutes you will spend reading this chapter will change your concept about what skin really is, how it works, and what "skin care" is all about. It will also bring the rest of this book into focus for you.

After talking with hundreds of women, and reading skin-care advertisements, I definitely get the idea that skin is just not understood. Somehow, skin is thought of as a substance like leather, to be treated accordingly—cleansed, polished, oiled, softened. Skin is a complex living organ, but it is made to take care of itself (and the rest of you inside it) with remarkably little help.

Think of facial skin as a three-layer structure: a tissue-paper-thin top layer called the stratum corneum, another very thin layer beneath it called the epidermis, and a much thicker layer beneath that called the dermis. Beneath the skin of the face is a thin layer of muscle tissue, which enables the face to assume its many expressions. Beneath the muscle layer is a thin layer of fat. To get a hands-on feeling for this, take a pinch of your facial skin between your thumb and forefinger—you are holding *two* layers of all of this. And notice the differences in thickness in various areas: the skin around the eyes (the

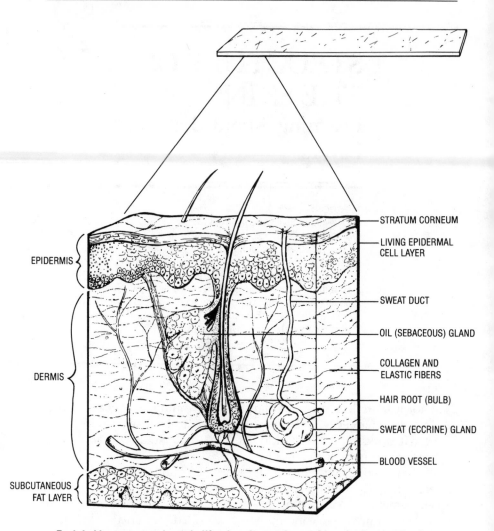

Facial skin: an approximately life-size view and an enlarged microscopic view.

STRATUM CORNEUM

LIVING EPIDERMAL CELL LAYER

SWEAT DUCT

OIL (SEBACEOUS) GLAND

COLLAGEN AND ELASTIC FIBERS

HAIR ROOT (BULB)

SWEAT (ECCRINE) GLAND

BLOOD VESSEL

EPIDERMIS

DERMIS

SUBCUTANEOUS FAT LAYER

eyelids and the skin above and below them) is very thin, the skin of the cheeks much thicker.

The skin is your largest organ. It is alive, full of tissue juices, blood vessels, nerves, and living cells—except for the very topmost layer, the stratum corneum. That thin layer is lifeless; the cells in it are the remains of once-living epidermal cells now flattened and glued together into a sheet or membrane. You can see this when skin "peels" after a sunburn.

THE STRATUM CORNEUM

This tissue-paper-thin topmost layer performs a most important function. It is the barrier between the living you and the outside world. It is a remarkable barrier—very little of anything can pass through it. The stratum corneum prevents tissue fluids and body chemicals from leaking out of us, and it prevents substances that come in contact with skin from getting inside us. Dirt, chemicals, germs, viruses, and essentially all cosmetic and skin-care product ingredients are kept outside where they belong.

Taking care of the stratum corneum is what most skin care is all about. We want it to look pretty and healthy because that is the part of skin that others see. The fact is, very little of what is applied to the stratum corneum can or does penetrate. Cosmetic and skin-care product advertising leads you to believe that the touted products can help, or rejuvenate, or rebuild your facial skin. Substitute "stratum corneum" for "skin" in these advertisements and you will get a truer picture of what the advertisements are really saying—that those products can alter the look and feel only of that thin, lifeless top layer.

The stratum corneum is about twenty cell layers thick (but those twenty cell layers are only as thick as paper). It is in a dynamic state—ever changing and renewing itself. The older cell plates are constantly being shed from the surface—washing, rubbing, and scrubbing remove millions each day. New cell plates are at the same time being added to the bottom of the stratum corneum. The stratum corneum is totally renewed and replaced every three to four weeks.

The stratum corneum likes water. A moist stratum corneum is flexible, smooth, and translucent. A dry stratum corneum is dull in appearance, flaky on the surface, and maybe crinkled by tiny lines.

THE EPIDERMIS

The epidermis is a thin layer of living cells just beneath the stratum corneum. Its main function is to manufacture the stratum corneum. Epidermal cells are born at the bottom or basal layer, move upward as they mature, lose their living juices, and finally flatten and become part of the stratum corneum membrane.

The epidermis is nourished by the blood vessels in the layer beneath it. It is important to remember that the epidermis is made up of *living* cells; therefore, it cannot be dry. The cells in it are as juicy as any other living cells in any other part of the body.

Pigment cells (melanocytes) are present in the epidermis. The pigment they produce (melanin) winds up inside epidermal cells. The function of pigment is to provide protection from ultraviolet light (sunlight) penetration. The amount, kind, and degree of dispersion of pigment all contribute to the color tone of an individual's skin. Sunlight (ultraviolet light) stimulates melanocytes to produce pigment, which is why skin becomes darker when exposed to sunlight. Very fair skin cannot produce enough pigment to prevent sunlight from injuring epidermal cells, which is why fair skin develops skin cancers so easily. Nor does fair skin have enough pigment to prevent sunlight from penetrating to the next deeper layer of skin, the dermis. That is why fair skin develops wrinkles, for wrinkles are caused by a dermis weakened and thinned by sun exposure.

THE DERMIS

This is the deepest layer of skin, and far and away the thickest and strongest layer. It is the strength and structure of skin. It is elastic and resilient, stretching to accommodate the movement of facial expressions and then returning to its original shape.

The dermis, too, is alive and juicy. It is made of collagen and elastin fibers woven together. Between and among the fibers are living cells and a gel substance composed of water and body chemicals. The dermis also contains blood vessels and nerves, hair follicles, oil glands, and sweat glands.

The dermis, because it is alive, repairs and renews itself. But, unlike the epidermis and stratum corneum, which are regenerated rapidly, repair and renewal in the dermis are very slow. This is important to remember, for damage to the dermis—and the thing that damages the dermis is sunlight—is, in practical terms, *permanent.*

Sunlight penetrates through stratum corneum and epidermis into the dermis especially easily in fair skin, which does not have adequate protective melanin pigment. Sunlight slowly destroys the dermis. When exposed to sunlight year after year, the dermis loses its strength and resilience and becomes thin and weak. It sags. Facial expressions throw facial skin into folds and creases. Sun-damaged dermis, because it has lost is resilience, becomes permanantly folded and creased—in other words, *wrinkled.*

Age plays a role here, too. In old age the dermis naturally becomes thinner and less strong. But the age factor does not significantly come into play until truly old age—not at thirty years.

The dermis does not ever become "dry." It is inside the body and always full of tissue juices. That is a simple statement that should be remembered when you read cosmetic and skin-care product advertisements. The dermis does not need moisturizers; moisturizers do not penetrate to the dermis. Wrinkles and lines are caused by sun damage in the dermis (and age later in life) and *not* by surface dryness.

More on the subjects of wrinkles and sun damage in chapters 3 and 8.

REVIEW

The first step in understanding facial skin care has been taken. You should now understand the structure of facial skin and something about how it works. Remember these key skin facts:

The *stratum corneum,* the tissue-paper-thin top layer of skin, is a barrier to loss of body fluids and to the penetration of external substances.

The stratum corneum is being made anew constantly by the *epidermis* beneath it. Epidermis is living tissue and never becomes dry. Sunlight damages epidermal cells, and that can result in skin cancers.

The *dermis* is the deepest and thickest layer of skin, giving skin its bulk, strength, elasticity, resilience, and contour. It is alive and juicy and never dry. It is damaged by sun exposure, which leads to wrinkles. The dermis is very slow to repair itself.

Skin-care efforts and products can make the stratum corneum look and feel softer but have little effect on the deeper layers of skin.

3

LINES, WRINKLES, AND CRINKLES
The Big Concern

QUESTION:
  What can I do about these wrinkles?
ANSWER:
  The first step is to understand the different kinds of wrinkles:
  expression lines, real wrinkles, and surface *crinkles.* The next
  step is to understand what skin care can and cannot do
  for these problems. This chapter is about what causes those
  different types of wrinkles.

This is an area of enormous concern to most women; it is also a subject that is misunderstood. Wrinkles and lines are equated with "aging." No one wants to look "old." Some women will go to any lengths to try to look younger, buying anything that promises to erase wrinkles and lines, and believing any cosmetic or skin-care-product advertising claim that promises to reverse the "aging process."

The makers of cosmetic and skin-care products, and those who are paid to create the advertising, do little to educate the public about aging, wrinkles, and lines. Instead, they take advantage of the fact that few women understand what wrinkles, lines, and crinkles are, why they have them, and what can realistically can be done about them.

Facial lines are divided here into three types in the hope that the "line" problem will be easier to understand. There is much overlapping among the three.

14

EXPRESSION LINES

Furrows in the brow, frown lines between the brows, smile lines on the cheeks around the mouth, and smile lines around the eyes are examples of expression lines. They come from a combination of habitual facial expressions and heredity. Yes, you can inherit the tendency for developing expression lines just as you can inherit nearly everything else.

Habitual facial expressions such as smiling, furrowing the brow, and frowning continually throw the skin into folds. With time and countless repetitions, the folds become permanent; the deeper layer of skin, the dermis, becomes forever creased.

Expression lines are more pronounced in sun-damaged skin, and become deeper with years. Sun damage and age cause the dermis to be less resilient, less able to snap back into shape after being thrown into a crease by the facial muscles. Smile lines around the eyes are certainly always a product of facial expression plus sun damage. The dermis is quite thin around the eyes and therefore is more easily damaged by the sun.

Facial expression lines develop in both dry and oily skins. As a matter of fact, expression lines are often more prominent in individuals who have oily skin. Dryness simply has little to do with facial expression lines. Therefore, moisturizers do not help expression lines (except in the area around the eyes, where the dermis is very thin). Stop frowning and start smiling. Expression lines from smiling are more flattering.

WRINKLES

Wrinkles are caused by ultraviolet light exposure and age. Ultraviolet exposure (from sunlight or artificial sources) damages the deeper layer of the skin (the dermis) and makes it thinner, less strong, less resilient, and saggy. The sags have to go somewhere, and the muscles of facial expression cause the sags to align themselves as wrinkles along the normal expression areas of the face.

The areas where wrinkles are most prominent are where skin is thinnest (around the eyes) and where most facial expression occurs (around the eyes and mouth).

Blonds and redheads wrinkle more and sooner than brunets. Blue- and green-eyed individuals wrinkle more and sooner than persons with darker eyes.

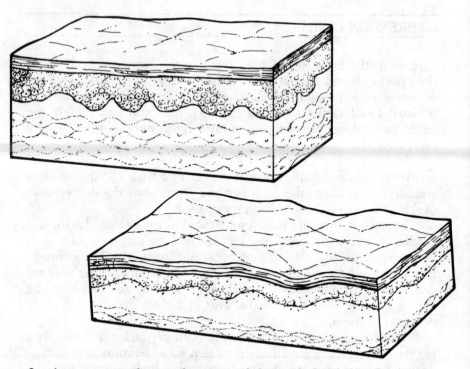

Sun damage causes degenerative *structural* changes in facial skin. *Top:* Healthy, young firm skin. *Bottom:* Sun-damaged, thin, weak, wrinkled skin.

Individuals with deeply pigmented skin (for example, East Indians) do not wrinkle much. Individuals with black skin wrinkle almost not at all. Why? Because deep color pigment in the skin protects the dermis from ultraviolet light, and it is ultraviolet light from sun exposure through the years that causes wrinkles. Age does play a role in wrinkling, but look at an old person with very dark or black skin and you will not see many wrinkles. Time is a factor, but *time in the sun* is a much bigger factor for the fair-skinned. It is that simple. And, to answer an often-asked question, time spent in tanning booths or beds is just as apt to cause wrinkles as time spent in the sun.

Wrinkle-causing sun damage starts as soon as the sun starts hitting the skin. In adult life enough sun damage may have accumulated so that wrinkles start appearing. If the dermis repairs itself from sun damage at all, it is extremely slow. Practically speaking, once the dermis is damaged by ultraviolet light exposure, it stays that way.

Darker-complected individuals may have to really work at getting enough sun or artifical ultraviolet light exposure to cause wrinkles. Fair-skinned individuals do not have to try hard at all—just the accidental sun exposure of daily life may be enough. Fair-skinned individuals who sunbathe or who are occupationally or recreationally exposed to lots of sun are going to get really wrinkled.

The key to avoiding wrinkles in those fair-skinned, wrinkle-prone faces is prevention of sun damage. It is important to understand that this *prevention must start at an early age and continue through life.* (See chapter 8.)

Remember, oily skin does *not* mean protection from wrinkles. Therefore moisturizers *cannot* significantly help to eliminate wrinkles, nor can they prevent wrinkles. Moisturizers do not penetrate into the skin deeper than the stratum corneum (top layer). Moisturizers can temporarily soften the appearance of *tiny* wrinkles to camouflage them, but make no real difference in the deeper ones. No matter what the cosmetic and skin-care advertisements imply or promise, there just is no magic skin-care product available now to repair sun-damaged dermis—to cure wrinkles—and that is a fact. But retinoic acid *may* prove to be the exception. (See chapter 7.)

"New miracle breakthroughs" to help "prevent the signs of aging," "repair overnight," "stimulate the skin circulation," "firm," and "lift" (all really referring to wrinkles) are being announced constantly—new ones each year, one after another. This fact in itself is an indication that last year's miracle breakthrough did not really work after all!

Those advertisements are nearly irresistible. They seem to promise so much. But right now there is nothing available in a bottle or jar from any cosmetics counter that will make a significant or lasting change in the weakened substance of skin.

But there is help—the kind dermatologists and plastic surgeons can give. Cosmetic surgery, skin peeling, and injections of collagen (Zyderm) into the skin all have their place in helping resurface, redrape, and/or reshape wrinkled facial skin.

Consult a dermatologist or plastic surgeon for help with wrinkles. Money spent with these professionals will result in far more significant help for skin lines than money spent at the cosmetics counter.

CRINKLES

This is the authors' term—used to describe the surface texture of facial skin when the stratum corneum is actually dry. Crinkles caused by dry skin are the same as the "tiny lines" referred to in skin-care product advertisements.

Crinkles show up because the stratum corneum shrinks a little when it is dry and, in so doing, pulls thin facial skin into tiny lines.

Crinkles are far more likely to appear in areas where the skin is thin and soft. The area around the eyes is particularly susceptible in everyone. Some individuals with naturally thin skin and sun damage get crinkles all over the face when the sun surface becomes dry.

So, whereas lines and wrinkles are a product of sun damage, heredity, and facial expressions, crinkles are primarily a product of surface dryness. Sun-damaged skin, because it is thinner and weaker, is more prone to crinkles, too, so there is a lot of overlap between crinkles and small wrinkles.

Crinkles *can* be helped by moisturizing skin-care products. Simple moisturizing swells stratum corneum cells and smooths out the top layer of skin. And this really does help crinkles disappear temporarily.

4

PORES
Can You Shrink Them?

QUESTION:

I have large pores in my face. Is there anything I can do to shrink them?

ANSWER:

There are some skin-care measures in this chapter that help pores *temporarily* appear smaller. But pore size is related to underlying oil gland size and is just a part of how your skin is made. There really is no way to permanently shrink pores—to change the way your skin is made.

Pores are openings in the skin's surface from which hairs grow and through which oil from oil glands flows to the surface. Everyone knows those things. But it seems few individuals understand some other simple facts about pores:

- that the size of a pore is proportional to the size of the oil gland under it
- that there is really *no* way to permanently "shrink" pores
- that many skin-care products and practices actually make pores appear larger

WHY SMALL PORES BECOME LARGE

Pores are small in infancy and childhood, simply because infants and children have very small facial oil glands. Remember, pore size is related to oil gland size.

At puberty, when the sex hormones begin to flow, oil glands get much larger very quickly. Pores enlarge to accommodate the increased oil flow, but often they can not enlarge as fast as oil glands do. So what happens? Acne: blackheads, whiteheads, and pimples. Small pores with large oil flow seem to get blocked easily, and that is where acne gets its start.

As pores enlarge enough to accommodate the oil flow, acne clears up. And that is most likely the reason why individuals tend to "outgrow" acne. Just how hormones control oil glands is not yet completely understood, but it is generally thought that sex hormones having male hormone characteristics are the ones that cause oil gland stimulation. Females also have male hormones; they are produced by the ovaries and the adrenal glands.

BIG PORES

If you have big pores, it simply means you have big oil glands and the pores have grown to a size necessary to accommodate the oil flow. If you were to *really* decrease pore size, you might develop acne! So if you don't have acne, stop thinking about shrinking pores—your pores are the appropriate size for your oil glands.

MAKING PORES APPEAR SMALLER

Although pores can't be permanently "shrunk," they can be made to appear smaller by appropriate skin-care measures.

The measures that can accomplish this, in general, are ones that remove moisture (water) from the stratum corneum. Stratum corneum cell plates swell when soaked with water and shrink when dried out. The diagram below shows how that affects the apparent size of pores.

The following are some specific suggestions for skin care that will make pores appear smaller. Some of these measures may be too harsh for your skin. Pick those that feel most appropriate to you.

Cleanse the skin well. Use plain bath soap, but not one that is moisturizing, creamy, or superfatted. Other cleansers labeled "for oily skin" are usually fine, too, as long as they *lather* and rinse away with water.

Use astringents or fresheners. These products contain alcohol, water, and some other cleansing agents. The ones specified for oily skin usually contain more alcohol and work best at making pores appear smaller. Alcohol helps remove water from stratum corneum cells, making them flatter and thereby making pores appear smaller.

Use "scrub" cleansers. Gently scrubbing with these removes the top stratum corneum cells and therefore reduces the thickness of that layer. That makes pores appear smaller.

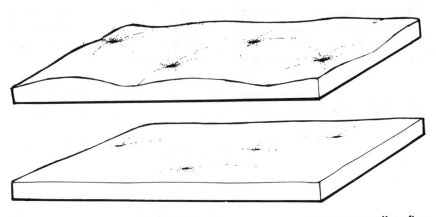

Top: **Large pores in facial skin.** *Bottom:* **The same pores now** *appear* **smaller after proper cleansing and the use of an astringent.**

Use cleansing pads or brushes. They do the same job as abrasive cleansers and have similar effects on pores.

Use cleansing masks. These products (particularly clay-based ones) reduce the amount of water in the stratum corneum and also remove some of the top layer of stratum corneum cells.

Do not moisturize. Never moisturize the areas of the face that have large pores. Moisturizing makes pores appear larger.

Use oil-absorbing foundation makeup. Any of those recommended for oily or acne-prone skin in chapter 12 will do nicely. They absorb skin oils and moisture from the surface and make pores appear smaller. The same goes for loose face powders. See specific camouflage tips in that chapter.

But what about skin dryness from all these measures to control pore size? Remember, big pores mean big oil glands and skin that is plenty oily. Drying out the stratum corneum some will not hurt the skin, it just makes pores appear smaller. You may prefer slight surface dryness to the big-pore look. You cannot have it both ways! Continual use of these skin-care measures will give you some control over pore size, but will not completely solve the problem.

BIG PORES AND DRY SKIN

If you have scaly, dry areas on your face but are confused because you also have big pores (which this book says means oily), you may have seborrheic dermatitis and should read chapter 15. A few individuals have a stratum corneum that is truly dry (doesn't hold water well) and tends to be flaky, but also have big pores and oily skin. In this rare case it is better to moisturize and tolerate the large pores.

BIG PORES AND WRINKLES

If you have facial wrinkles and dry skin, but are confused by the fact that you also have big pores, reread chapter 3.

DRY SKIN

5

QUESTION:
   If my facial skin feels rough and flaky, it means I have dry skin, right?

ANSWER:
   Maybe yes, maybe no. There is a very common skin problem called seborrheic dermatitis that can cause facial skin to feel rough and dry in places. The paradox is that seborrheic dermatitis occurs only on oily faces. If you have those rough dry facial areas, be sure to read chapter 15, "Seborrheic Dermatitis," before you buy a new, expensive moisturizer; perhaps you should buy an *inexpensive* *medicine* instead.

The magnitude of the concern, the time, the advertising, and the dollars spent on what is perceived as the dry-skin problem is truly astounding. It is matched by the magnitude of the misunderstanding of this problem.

The American public spends $500 *million* per year on moisturizers alone. Is dry skin truly epidemic, or is it a myth of major proportions?

Frankly, the odds are that your *facial* skin is not as "dry" as you may think. Understanding the question of dry skin is a key to understanding skin care. If you want to take good sensible care of your skin and not be duped by cosmetic and skin-care-product claims and sales pitches, it is essential that you understand "dry skin."

Many of the dermatologists I know are astounded by the numbers of women consulting them who have obvious signs of oily skin (large pores, blackheads, acne breakouts, oily hair, and seborrheic dermatitis) and still persist in the notion that they have dry skin. Why? Because they have some wrinkles and lines, or because they feel a little tight and "dry" after washing their faces. Neither of these is necessarily a sign of dry skin. The cosmetic and skin-care industry simply has the female public so thoroughly indoctrinated toward thinking "dry" that it seems very few women are able to look at their faces with any objectivity.

Some misconceptions about dry skin:

We all have it. Skin-care advertisements and most skin-care experts tell everyone that they have dry skin and need moisturizing. That's not so.

Wrinkles mean skin is dry; wrinkles result from dry skin. These have to be the most common misconceptions of all. Wrinkles really have little or nothing to do with skin dryness, nor does moisturizing help or prevent wrinkles. Read chapter 3, "Lines, Wrinkles, and Crinkles," so you will understand about this.

Flaking and scaling are signs of dryness. These problems may be a sign of dermatitis (irritated skin), especially seborrheic dermatitis. If you have flaking facial skin areas but also large pores and oily areas, be sure to read chapter 15, "Seborrheic Dermatitis."

WHAT DRY SKIN REALLY IS

Skin dryness is a lack of *water* in the paper-thin, nonliving top layer of skin, the stratum corneum. Dryness does not affect the deeper layers of skin, the living epidermis and dermis. These deeper layers are living tissue; they are "inside" the body; they are constantly bathed in tissue fluids; and they are never "dry." It is so important to understand this. These deeper layers make up more than 80 percent of the skin's thickness and strength, and they are *always* moist and plump. Deterioration and weakening of the dermis from sun exposure and time are the causes of wrinkles. Even deteriorated dermis stays moist all the time. Wrinkles are not a sign of dry skin.

So the stratum corneum is the only part of skin that can be dry. Let us take a closer look at that layer.

The stratum corneum is very thin—a good deal thinner than the paper this book is printed on. It is made of dead epidermal cells, flattened into plates and glued together into a sheet, or membrane, by intercellular substance. The uppermost cells are constantly leaving us—being washed off and rubbed off daily. New stratum corneum cell plates are at the same time being added to the lower layers of the stratum corneum. The stratum corneum is, therefore, a dynamic layer—being lost and replenished constantly. In this ongoing process, the entire layer is replaced every three weeks or so.

When the stratum corneum is dry (lacking water), it is stiff, rough or flaky, crinkly, and dull in appearance. Under a microscope dry stratum corneum cell plates look like corn flakes, brittle and rough. Dry stratum corneum shrinks a little, pulling thin skin into tiny lines (crinkles, but not wrinkles).

When the stratum corneum is moist (full of water), it is flexible, smooth, and translucent. Microscopically, the surface is smoother and less irregular, more like a shingled roof. When moist with water, stratum corneum cell plates swell and plump up, easing the surface into smoothness—easing away crinkles (but having no effect on real wrinkles).

Please notice there has been no mention of oil in softening or moisturizing stratum corneum, though we often think of oil or grease when we think of moisturizing. Actually, oil does not soak into stratum corneum at all; it only lies on the surface. Water is what the stratum corneum needs to be moist; oil can only serve to help keep water in the stratum corneum.

The stratum corneum becomes dry for several reasons. First, our skins are not all made alike. The ability of the stratum corneum to hold water varies from individual to individual. Likewise, the ability of the stratum corneum cell plates and the intercellular substance to hold together as an intact membrane varies. Second, the skin oils produced by the oil glands vary in amount and composition from individual to individual. The main purpose of skin oil is to coat the surface of the stratum corneum to keep moisture (water) in the stratum corneum. In general, individuals who produce more skin oil have less trouble with surface dryness. There are those fairly rare persons who have plenty of skin oil but have a stratum corneum that does not hold water well or hold together well. They get "dry" in spite of being "oily." Third, the humidity of the environment plays a major role in surface skin dryness. When humidity is high, over 60 percent, the stratum corneum cells stay moist; there is enough water in the air to keep them from drying so much. When the humidity is low, under 60 percent, the stratum corneum tends to lose its water to the air, and therefore becomes dry faster and more easily. Low humidity is a problem for skin year-round in some arid climates. It is a very big problem in colder climates, where heated indoor air may have *very* low humidity. Fourth, improper skin cleansing and frequent repeated wetting and drying of the stratum corneum can create dry-skin problems. Water and many cleansing agents tend to dissolve away the intercellular substance of the stratum corneum (the glue that holds the stratum corneum cells together) and even tends to damage the stratum corneum cells themselves. These factors lead to increased surface dryness. Good cleansing is always important, but delicate, easily-dried-out skin needs to be cleansed more gently than skin that is not so delicate. There has to be a balance struck between cleansing that is thorough enough for the individual skin type and cleansing that is too harsh. And that balance varies much from individual to individual. (See chapter 9, "Daily Cleansing—The Simple, Inexpensive Way.")

AGE AND DRY SKIN

This is an area in which the cosmetic and skin-care industry has the public confused. You are told that dryness is a sign of aging, that if you are aging you have dry skin, that moisturizing stops the "signs of aging," and that (usually implied, not said) you can prevent or cure the signs of aging by using moisturizers and other skin-care products.

Some of this is true, if you understand that wrinkles are a sign of sun damage and *not* of dry skin, and that the effects of age insofar as dry skin is concerned do not occur significantly until middle age (over fifty years). But no skin-care product can prevent aging of the skin. Sunblocking products can help prevent sun damage, but they do nothing to prevent the changes that come naturally with age. See chapter 8, "Sun Damage—Sun Protection."

Here is what we do know about age and skin dryness:

As time passes, the stratum corneum does seem to get drier—to lose its water-holding ability. The rate of turnover of the living epidermis slows down some, and therefore the rate at which the stratum corneum is manufactured is slowed. The lifeless stratum corneum cells stay on the skin surface longer; in doing so, they dry out more.

When does this happen? It happens gradually through life, but the effects of age on the stratum corneum do not really show up significantly until pretty late in life—after fifty years or so. Beyond fifty (but this varies greatly) more profound changes occur in *all* layers of the skin—even the living epidermis and dermis. The whole skin becomes weaker, thinner, and much less resilient.

In summary, age does play a role in dryness of skin but not until later in life, around age fifty, and not at age thirty, when you are being told it does. The fact is that many women around the age of thirty begin to see the effects of sun damage (small wrinkles and lines), but their skin is no drier than it was ten years earlier. In fact, many women at around age thirty seem to be producing *more* skin oil than they did ten years earlier.

COMBINATION SKIN

"Combination skin" is an often-used phrase, and the truth is that *everyone* has skin that is somewhat oilier in the "T" zone, which consists of the forehead and middle third of the face. (See chapter 6, "Oily Skin," page 29, for a treatment for this condition.) In some individuals that difference is more noticeable than in others. Many cases of so-called combination skin are actually oily faces with patches of seborrheic dermatitis. If you think you have "combination skin," be sure to read Chapter 15, "Seborrheic Dermatitis."

SKIN THAT FEELS TIGHT OR DRY AFTER WASHING

This sensation is simply normal. It does not necessarily mean that you have dry skin; plenty of individuals with oily skin also experience it. Skin can be delicate or a little sensitive without being dry.

If this feeling of tightness really is a bother, there are several solutions. Wait thirty minutes and the sensation will pass. Use gentler cleansers. Apply a very light moisturizer just after washing. If your face feels *really* sensitive after washing, it may be a sign of seborrheic dermatitis or another form of dermatitis or eczema.

WHAT TO DO ABOUT DRY SKIN

Now that we are all convinced that water is what the stratum corneum needs to keep it smooth, flexible, and pretty, it seems only logical that keeping water there is what we need to do. And so, the simple secret to moisturizing is revealed: Get water into the stratum corneum and keep it there by putting something on top that will not let water evaporate.

Most moisturizing products contain water and some kind of oil. The water soaks into the stratum corneum cells and thereby does the "moisturizing." The oil stays on the surface and helps keep the water in the stratum corneum.

There are thousands of formulations for moisturizers, and some are better than others. Though they have different smells and textures, they all work in basically the same way—regardless of the wide variation in price and the outlandish claims that are made for some of them.

Some moisturizers do not contain water, just an oil of some kind. They work by trapping water that seeps into the stratum corneum through sweat glands.

Some moisturizers contain "special ingredients." These are discussed in chapter 11, "Moisturizing."

THE LAST WORDS

You are almost certainly a consumer of "dry skin" products. It is hoped that now you are an educated consumer and understand what dry skin is and what it is not, what moisturizers can do and what they cannot do.

If you have a dry stratum corneum, seasonally or all the time, use moisturizers. Pay no more for them than you want to, for there is as little magic in moisturizers as there is mystery in dry skin.

OILY SKIN

QUESTION:
> I have oily skin. That will keep me from having wrinkles, won't it?

ANSWER:
> The development of wrinkles depends much more on skin, hair, and eye color, and on the amount of sun exposure, than on whether skin is oily. In general, individuals with oily skin are somewhat darker in skin tone than those with nonoily skin—that that helps some in preventing wrinkles. But there are plenty of oily-skinned individuals around who are quite wrinkled.

You would hardly know it from reading cosmetic and skin-care advertisements, but many women have oily skin. Maybe just a little oily, maybe very oily. Most women with very oily skin know it; most women with slightly to moderately oily skin do not. They have been so thoroughly persuaded to think that their skin is dry that they completely overlook the fact that they have oily facial skin.

WHY OILY SKIN

In infancy and childhood, facial oil glands are very small and do not produce much oil. At puberty, when hormones start flowing, oil glands become much larger and produce more oil. How large oil glands become and how much oil is produced depend on two factors: (1) the amount and kind of hormones produced and (2) the genetic determination of the individual.

In recent years, significant attention has been focused on researching the amount and types of hormones and how they affect oil gland size and activity. The understanding of hormonal control of oil glands is incomplete, but, speaking generally, male hormones stimulate oil glands. Male hormones in women are produced by both the ovaries and the adrenal glands. The total amount of, and types of, an individual's hormones directly affects the oiliness of facial skin.

29

The genetic determination factor is simple to explain. Just as nearly every other characteristic of an individual is inherited, so is the tendency to oily skin. If one parent has oily skin, each child has about a fifty-fifty chance of being born with the tendency to oily skin. If both parents have oily skin, each child has a nearly 100 percent chance of developing oily skin.

SIGNS OF OILY SKIN

Large pores. They indicate that there are large oil glands under them.

Oily hair. Hair that needs frequent shampooing means oily facial skin.

Blackheads and whiteheads.

Acne breakouts.

Seborrheic dermatitis of the scalp and face.

Oily appearance and feel, sometimes only an hour after washing the face.

DEALING WITH OILY SKIN

Some women with very oily skin have an excess amount of hormones that are responsible for overstimulating the facial oil glands. However, most women are hormonally in perfect balance and simply have oily skin.

Hormone excess may come from the ovaries or the adrenal glands. Blood tests can be done to determine if hormone excess is the cause of extra oiliness, and whether the excess is coming from the ovaries or the adrenal glands. Those individuals with extra-oily skin may want to consult with a dermatologist or endocrinologist about having those tests done. Let your physician advise you here about whether the tests really need to be done and whether the required hormone-balancing treatment would be appropriate for you.

There is research in progress now searching for a safe and effective way to control oil gland secretions. The ideal product would be effective when applied topically to oily areas. Such a product is not yet available to us. Until a really good solution to the problem of extra-oily skin comes along, you must rely on skin-care techniques that can keep the problem manageable:

Cleansing should be rigorous and frequent. This removes oil and dead skin cells that build up on oily skin. Oily skin can look dull if this buildup is not removed. Use cleansing masks, scrubbing cleansers, and scrubbing pads or sponges. Soaps and cleansers for oily skin are recommended. Inexpensive bath soaps, such as Ivory, work as well. Liquid detergent skin cleansers such as Phisoderm are perhaps the best of all for removing skin oils.

Astringents also help. Use the kind labeled "for oily skin." They help remove oil and dead skin cells, and they make pores appear smaller.

Makeup foundation should be a "matte" type. Read chapter 12 for specific suggestions.

Loose powder helps blot and absorb excess skin oils.

Controlling lotions sold by some cosmetic lines help control the oily look when applied before the makeup foundation. Try Aller-creme's Oil Regulating Lotion, Germaine Monteil's Under Makeup Toner, and Erno Laslo's Conditioning Preparation.

OILY SKIN THAT IS ALSO DRY OR SENSITIVE

This is a problem that needs some understanding. Some women have some of the above signs of oily skin but are confused by (1) the feeling of dryness or tightness after bathing the face and (2) flaking or scaling areas of the face.

In the first case, the feeling of dryness or tightness after bathing the face is normal in many individuals. It may also mean that the facial skin is sensitive, and perhaps that the cleansing routine is too harsh. Sensitivity may come from a tendency to seborrheic dermatitis or atopic eczema (allergic eczema). Or you may just have sensitive facial skin.

In the second case, flaking or scaling areas of the face are most probably caused by seborrheic dermatitis. Suspect this especially if the flaking areas are on the brows and forehead, around the nose, ears, or hairline, and if you have a flaky or itchy scalp. Another cause of flaking facial skin is allergic (atopic) eczema. A family or personal history of asthma and hay fever or a history of childhood eczema can be the tip-off here. Individuals who have problems with eczema or dermatitis elsewhere (especially of the hands) also tend to have facial skin that develops scaly areas with the slightest irritation.

For help in dealing with this tricky skin situation, try some of the following suggestions:

1. Use gentle cleansing methods, but do not skip the use of a lathering cleanser. Read chapter 9, "Daily Cleansing."

2. Use a very light moisturizer after cleansing. There are several "oil-free" moisturizers available that are good choices for oily but

sensitive skin. Try Clarifiance by Lancôme. Less expensive are Wibi Lotion and Cetaphil Lotion (the cream form of Cetaphil is better—ask a pharmacist for it).

Be careful of any moisturizer on facial areas prone to acne breakouts. Any of them may increase the chances of breakouts.

3. Hydrocortisone creams (the kind you can buy without a doctor's prescription) are quite effective for calming irritated facial skin. Use these products after cleansing if you are troubled with more than just a little irritation after cleansing. They are especially useful in cases of facial dermatitis or eczema. But these products are *not safe for prolonged use.* Read the package insert.

4. Read chapter 15, "Seborrheic Dermatitis." If you think you have this problem, try some of the treatment routines suggested.

PART TWO

SKIN
CARE

7

ADVERTISING CLAIMS, SPECIAL INGREDIENTS, LABELING, AND SKIN REJUVENATION

QUESTION:
> If the new advanced skin-care products cannot really do what the advertisements say, why are the cosmetics companies allowed to advertise as they do?

ANSWER:
> Those advertisements are worded so skillfully that they seem to promise more than they really do. Only the most well-informed reader is equipped to see through these advertisements. The Federal Trade Commission and the Food and Drug Administration are protecting the public's health and safety quite well, but they are not doing much to protect our gullibility and our pocketbooks.

ADVERTISING CLAIMS

Reading cosmetics ads gives one the impression that modern skin-care products can really change facial skin—that whatever the facial skin problem, it can surely be cured by these new highly scientific products.

We tend to believe what we *read* anywhere. We believe what we read in cosmetics advertisements because they are so well and attractively done, maybe because we feel that our laws ensure that advertising claims are truthful, because high tech is "in" (those ads certainly sound scientific and technical), and because we all want to believe that something can make us look more youthful and beautiful. Have you ever noticed how attractive and young most of the models are in these ads? It's just too easy for a consumer to get the message that her skin could look like a model's by using these products.

But are those advertising promises kept? Has our skin really changed after using the latest "miracle" product? Or have we been lured into spending time and money only to see the same wrinkles? Think about these questions.

The truth is that no *cosmetic* product can really remove or prevent wrinkles. Neither can it reverse or, practically speaking, prevent the "signs of aging." (There is a prescription medicine, retinoic acid, that may help—more about that below.)

This chapter is for anyone who would like to understand more about how misleading cosmetic and skin-care product advertising can be, about what those "miracle" ingredients can and cannot do, and about the real meaning (or lack thereof) of some product-labeling words.

FEDERAL REGULATORY AGENCIES AND COSMETICS ADVERTISING

There are two government agencies that have a role in regulating the advertisements you read: the Federal Trade Commission (FTC), which has responsibility for truth in advertising, and the Food and Drug Administration (FDA), which has responsibility for the purity and safety of cosmetics and for the safety, efficacy, and claims made for drugs.

Federal Trade Commission

Though the FTC has responsibility for truth in advertising, it does not approve advertisements before you see them. This means that cosmetics makers may say anything they wish about one of their products, true or not, without any require prior approval. Only when an advertising claim is blatantly false or when complaints are filed does the FTC take an interest.

The legal process is so costly and time-consuming that the FTC simply does not pursue misleading advertising claims unless it perceives that a claim is blatant and/or that the consumer can be significantly harmed by the claim. This state of affairs in the present system of regulating advertising has led to exactly what we see in cosmetics advertising—claims that are false or vague but worded so cleverly that they are difficult to pin down as false. A cosmetics maker can make untrue advertising claims—within limits—and simply get away with it.

Food and Drug Administration

The FDA has the responsibility of assuring the purity and safety of cosmetic products. Its regulations, along with the specter of legal action by consumers (the maker of a product that harms consumers will get sued!), has ensured a high level of safety in cosmetics. To be sure, there have been a few problem products, but on the whole the record has been a good one.

Another major responsibility of the FDA is regulating *drugs*—among other things, their manufacture and claims for their safety and efficacy.

Drugs are defined as substances that can cure an illness or alter the structure, function, or physiology of an organ—in this case, skin. Cosmetics, on the other hand, just make skin *look* prettier or different. There is some overlap here, but the difference is clear—drugs can significantly change skin, cosmetics cannot.

Many new skin-care products are advertised as though they have the effects of drugs—claiming to change, stimulate, rebuild, or otherwise truly alter skin. Yet essentially none of those products so advertised has the approval of the FDA as a drug! (Sunblock ingredients are the exception, for these substances are classified as drugs.)

As to how cosmetics makers can get away with advertising *cosmetic* products with *drug* effects, the situation is much like that with the FTC. That is, the FDA simply does not have the time, staff, or money to pursue those makers—unless, that is, the FDA perceives a situation to be a blatant violation of regulations or a health hazard to consumers.

But the truth is that if a cosmetic product or ingredient had druglike effects of any consequence (can really alter the structure, function, or physiology of skin), then the sale or promotion of that product or ingredient without FDA drug approval could be considered *illegal*. On the other hand, if a product or ingredient does not have the druglike effects it claims, then those claims are false!

Claims made in many cosmetic and skin-care product advertisements often seem to point toward one or the other of the above situations.

FDA note: In the spring of 1987, the FDA sent regulatory letters to twenty-two major cosmetics manufacturers challenging their claims made for, and their labeling of skin-care products. These challenges were aimed at the making of "drug-type" claims for products that did not have FDA approval as drugs. Claims such as "antiaging," "rejuvenation," and "cell renewal" indicate that the intended use of a *cosmetic* product is to alter the structure and function of skin, not just to beautify it. And, that's against FDA regulations.

Apparently getting less than the desired response from cosmetics makers, another letter, stronger in intent, was sent by the FDA in the spring of 1988. This letter threatened injunction and even seizure of cosmetic products.

This should be welcome news to consumers. Our federal regulatory agencies have always tried to do a creditable job in protecting our health and safety, now we see them protecting our gullibility and our pocketbooks.

Vanity and the never-ending search for youth and beauty make us so susceptible to promises of hope. You can, however, become an informed consumer—more skeptical about what you read, more realistic in your expectations, and able to use your own knowledge to care very well for your skin.

SPECIAL INGREDIENTS

There are quite a few "special ingredients" in cosmetic and skin-care products to add "special" properties to them. They also lend themselves to advertising claims. The following sections describe some of the more commonly used ones and what they can and cannot do for your skin.

Protein

Various proteins are added to many products to make you think they can help nourish your skin. Protein does not penetrate the stratum corneum, so it cannot nourish the skin. Some proteins can form a water-holding gel on the skin surface and therefore enhance the moisturizing properties of a product.

Collagen

Since the main structural protein of the dermis is collagen, and since sun-damaged wrinkled skin has a weak dermis, the hope is that you will believe that the collagen in a skin-care product will penetrate into and rebuild your dermis. One cosmetic line calls its collagen cream something like "sub skin" cream. Others allude to "firming" action, etc. Collagen in skin creams or liquids, whether just "collagen," "hydrolyzed collagen," or "procollagen," does *not* penetrate into the dermis and therefore cannot rebuild the dermis.

Collagen, like protein, *can* form a gel with water. The addition of collagen to a cosmetic product can help hold water on the skin surface by forming this gel film. Collagen is an inexpensive ingredient, but usually adds lots to the price of a product. If it feels good, use it. Just don't think it will help permanently rebuild or firm your skin. It will not.

Elastin

This skin-care product ingredient can be thought of in exactly the same way as collagen. It does not penetrate skin or make it more "elastic," though it can enhance the moisturizing properties of a product.

Aloe Vera

The juice of this cactuslike plant is credited with all sorts of miraculous healing powers. Though there is very scant scientific evidence that aloe really works any magic at all, it has such a huge following of believers that some cosmetics lines are capitalizing on it. The addition of aloe to cosmetic and skin-care products creates a significant market among the aloe believers. There is no evidence of particular benefits from using cosmetic and skin-care products that contain aloe.

Sunscreens

Dermatologists are in favor of adding sunscreens to cosmetic and skin-care products. Claims that products that contain a sunscreen "retard aging" are justified only if those products provide good protection (at least an SPF of 15). Most are not labeled with an SPF number, however. Such products will retard aging only if they are used continuously over a long period of time. The addition of sunscreens is a good thing, but do not be too taken in by those claims until you have read chapter 8. The claim "retards aging" is simply not justified by the addition of a small portion of a low-SPF sunscreen ingredient to a skin-care product.

Herbs, Fruits, Nuts, Vegetables, and Oils with Funny Names

All these and more are added to various skin-care products. They make good copy. Why, they sound good enough to eat. Though the addition of these ingredients would seem to be a good idea—helping to "nourish" facial skin—the fact is that little of what is in a cosmetic or skin-care product can penetrate to living cells. There seems to be little harm and little real help in using cosmetic products with such ingredients.

If the idea of "natural" or "organic" products is appealing to you, use them.

Vitamins

There have been and will continue to be skin-care products that claim beneficial effects because they contain vitamins. It sounds like a good idea, so it makes good advertising copy. There is little real evidence that gives credence to such claims.

Vitamin A is claimed to speed epidermal cell turnover rate when applied topically, so it may be promoted as a "cell renewal" stimulant.

Vitamin E is claimed to have extra moisturizing effects and even to help retard aging because of its antioxidant effects and its ability to neutralize free radicals (toxic metabolic chemicals). There is currently no definitive evidence that incorporating vitamin E into a skin-care product can significantly help skin. There *is* real evidence that some forms of vitamin E may cause severe allergies when applied to the skin. (Some of you who have broken open a capsule and applied it to your skin have learned the hard way.)

Phospholipids, Lecithin

These substances have the ability to bind numerous water molecules to each molecule of themselves. When added to moisturizing products, they may help hold water on the skin surface and therefore enhance the moisturizing effect.

Lactic Acid, Glycolic Acid, Urea

These substances are significant additives to moisturizing agents. They help bind water to the skin surface and also help remove dead skin cells. Removal of those dead cells makes skin feel and look smoother and softer. These ingredients can also cause a stinging sensation, and so they are used mainly in body moisturizers, not facial ones. At least one "overnight" face cream that contains urea is being marketed now. Urea will not make your skin young again, but the fact (technically correct) that urea does help remove dead surface skin cells gives rise to advertising that makes you *think* it will make your skin look young again!

Glycoprotein, Hyaluronic Acid, Chondrotin Sulfate, Mucopolysaccharides, Glycosphingolipid

Here again we have ingredients that are added to many of the new or high-tech skin-care products. These ingredients, like others we have discussed, help bind water and thus help keep the skin surface moist. These are the moisturizer boosters. They do not significantly penetrate into the deeper layers of the skin and cannot help rebuild skin.

Liposomes

At this writing, the latest high-tech cosmetic buzzword is "liposome." A liposome is basically a type of delivery system: It involves the encapsulation of a cosmetic ingredient—a mineral, a protein, a biologically active substance—into microscopically small droplets. These droplets have the ability to penetrate further into the stratum corneum, thereby acting as aids to the penetration of cosmetic ingredients.

Cosmetic products containing liposomes are selling quite well. Do liposomes make cosmetics, moisturizers, and antiaging creams work that much better, or is it just that the latest scientific discovery always enjoys brisk sales?

You should remember two things (they've been said before):

1. The penetration of cosmetic ingredients into the thin, non-living stratum corneum does *not* mean that such cosmetics can have a significant effect on the deeper and much thicker living layers of skin. Delivering, say, collagen deep within the skin does not guarantee that it will be integrated into the cell membranes or become biologically active.

2. By law, cosmetic ingredients may make skin look prettier, but they cannot alter the real structure, function, or physiology of living skin. Only ingredients that have been approved as *drugs* by the FDA can do those things.

Hormones

The addition of hormones—usually the female hormone estrogen—to moisturizing products is not new. It was in vogue a decade or more ago. Moisturizing products containing hormones are still available, but no longer heavily advertised. It is a nice idea—trying to feed aging skin the hormones of youth—but it just doesn't work significantly.

There is only a very small amount of hormone in these products, because adding more might cause enough hormone absorption through the skin to produce unwanted effects on the whole body.

LABELING

Hypoallergenic

This word means that a product so labeled does not produce many allergic reactions. That is to say, when tested on the skins of a group of individuals, few of them develop allergic rashes.

The word "hypoallergenic" has little meaning in describing modern cosmetic and skin-care products. The fact is that essentially all products from all reputable cosmetics makers are well tested for allergic potential before they are marketed. This testing is in the interest of the manufacturer as well as the consumer. No manufacturer wants to market a product that causes many allergic reactions.

So do not pay much attention to the label "hypoallergenic." Most cosmetic and skin-care products are in fact hypoallergenic and safe for almost everyone. Some allergic reactions do occur with every product, no matter how well tested.

"Hypoallergenic" does *not* mean that a cosmetic or skin-care product is unlikely to cause blocked pores, blackheads, whiteheads, and acne breakouts.

"Noncomedogenic"

This is a phrase dermatologists and some cosmetics makers have been talking about for years. At the time of this writing, this phrase is just beginning to be seen in cosmetic and skin-care labels and advertising copy.

"Noncomedogenic" means that a product will not cause comedones (blackheads or blocked pores). The purpose of this word is to imply that a particular product will not cause blocked pores or acne breakout problems and will not aggravate preexisting problems.

"Noncomedogenic" is even more difficult for the public to interpret properly than "hypoallergenic." The following should be clearly understood:

There is no FDA regulatory definition of "noncomedogenic," nor is there an industry standard for comedogenicity testing. Some manufacturers test for comedogenicity of a product, others do not. The tests are done on animals, seldom on people. The usual test model is the inside of a rabbit's ear. If a product can be applied to the skin inside the rabbit's ear for a few weeks without causing blocked pores, it will be certified "noncomedogenic."

This test is the best available in terms of cost, practicality, and meaningfulness, but it simply does not tell the whole story. The fact that a product passed this test means that at least the maker is trying to give you a product that will not cause or aggravate acne, and we should be grateful for this effort.

The fact remains that products labeled "noncomedogenic" may still cause or aggravate blackheads, blocked pores, and acne breakout problems in susceptible individuals. Sometimes it takes months of use before the bad effects appear.

So be wary of this label. Some dermatologists are interested enough in the role of cosmetic and skin-care products in acne that they can give you advice about products that, in their experience, have proven safe.

Unfortunately, the attempts of some researchers and cosmetics manufacturers to give real meaning to the term "noncomedogenic" are already being diluted by those who write ad copy. "Noncomedogenic" is becoming an important advertising buzzword. And, as those things go, it may become another tool to sell products to consumers rather than help them.

Hypoacnegenic, Nonacnegenic

These terms have much the same meaning as "noncomedogenic," with the emphasis more on not causing acne breakouts than on not causing blocked pores and blackheads. Again, there are no FDA regulatory definitions or industry standards for these words. The use of them in labeling and advertising means that the manufacturer has done some testing of the product. The significance is about the same as that of "noncomedogenic."

Deeply Penetrating

Many skin-care products use this claim in one way or another. It is misleading, in that very little of what is in a cosmetic or skin-care product can penetrate skin deeper than the stratum corneum (see chapter 2). The stratum corneum is made up of several layers of lifeless epidermal cell plates. When a product claims to penetrate "several layers of skin" or "to the deepest layer," it is only claiming to penetrate into a few layers of the stratum corneum, not into the living epidermis and dermis.

Firming and Lifting

These words are often used to give the consumer the impression that a product will act to do just that—whether it be a "treatment," a mask, or whatever. It should be understood that whatever happens will be more a feeling one gets from using a product than a reality. Any "firming" or "lifting" created by a cosmetic product is strictly temporary.

Unscented, Fragrance-Free

Again, these terms have no FDA regulatory definition. In general, "unscented" means "no perfume added" (perfumes are derived from natural vegetable and flower oils). But, an unscented product may contain a fragrance (an artificial sweet-smelling substance) to mask the unpleasant odor of cosmetic ingredients. Perfumes (scents) are frequently the culprit in allergic reactions to cosmetic and skin-care products. Fragrances cause problems, too, but less often than scents.

For those individuals sensitive to perfumes and scents, products labeled "unscented" are recommended. Even better are products labeled "unscented and fragrance-free."

SKIN REJUVENATION

Making skin look young again; retarding, diminishing, removing the "signs of aging," stimulating cell renewal, skin regeneration, and skin repair—these are the great chants of cosmetic and skin-care product makers and advertisers. Looking younger seems to be what we all want. We would love to be able to buy a product at the cosmetics counter that would accomplish this.

Consumers need to be skeptical about products that make such claims. Too many have spent too much only to discover that promises of "rebuilt" skin and a younger look just simply are not kept.

The following section discusses some of the claims and products and helps you to understand how they work and may not work. Included is retinoic acid (Retin A, tretinoin, vitamin A acid), which is a prescription medicine that really may help rejuvenate aged and sun-damaged skin.

Cellular, Stabilized Cell, Cell Extracts, Etc.

These usually come from some elite-sounding Swiss or French "institute." They are the most expensive of all the skin-care products. Although they make the advertising copy so appealing with intimations that these "cellular" extracts from embryos and placentas can "nourish" and "replenish" your skin, "challenge the aging process," etc., there is no evidence that they significantly help your skin. Their exorbitant prices are part of the marketing plan—anything that costs that much (sometimes a hundred dollars an ounce) *must* be good!

Overnight Repair, Cell-Renewal Stimulants

Cosmetics makers have certainly capitalized on this not-so-new idea. Old skin does have a slightly slower epidermal cell turnover rate than young skin. The addition of irritant chemicals to cosmetic products can step up the epidermal cell-renewal rate. And so, it is hoped, you will believe you are combating the aging of your skin by using these products. There is no evidence that your skin will significantly change with the use of these sometimes quite expensive products.

If you think skin stimulation and stepped-up epidermal cell renewal can do you some good, you can accomplish the same effects by scrubbing the skin, using granular scrub cleansers or facial cleansing sponges. You will not see claims of increased cell renewal attached to these old workhorse products because the advertisers want you to buy the newer, more expensive cell-renewal stimulants. Scrubbing cleansers and buffing sponges are actually better than cell-renewal creams, for they are extremely effective at removing dead skin cells and making the skin look brighter.

Skin Circulation Stimulants

This is another new thing in skin care—stimulating the blood circulation in the deepest layer of skin, the dermis. Although it sounds like an important thing, there is little evidence that stimulating skin circulation will significantly change your skin. Skin circulation, like epidermal cell turnover rate, can be stimulated by the use of scrubbing granular cleansers and facial cleansing or buffing sponges. Guess what causes that pink look your skin has after scrubbing? Yes, increased blood circulation!

Ampoules, Concentrates, Serums

These are usually small bottles with a distinctly "medical" look and a large price tag. They contain some advertised "concentrate," elixir, or "serum." They are usually sold to be used monthly or so, and are heralded by some really great-sounding advertising copy. Whether they contain collagen or cell-renewal stimulants or whatever, they prove that you can get a large amount of hype in a very small bottle.

Retinoic Acid (Retin A, Tretinoic, Vitamin A Acid)

Retinoic acid is a prescription drug that has been around a long time. When applied to the skin, it is an effective acne medication, and it has been used for this purpose for years. Recently, it has been scientifically shown to have significant biological effects on skin—the kind of effects that really may, to a degree, "rejuvenate" skin and slow down the "aging process."

But before you rush out and ask your doctor to prescribe retinoic acid for you, understand what is involved in its use. Improperly used, retinoic acid can cause redness, peeling, and itching. It is an irritant and is sometimes very tricky to use properly.

Retinoic acid can *quickly* help stimulate epidermal cell turnover rate, make the stratum corneum thinner and more translucent, help unblock blocked pores, improve skin circulation, and give facial skin a rosy, healthy glow.

Retinoic acid can *very slowly* help even out skin pigment tone, help remove precancerous lesions, cause the growth of new blood vessels in the skin, and stimulate the formation of new collagen support fibers in the dermis.

Sounds wonderful? Is this the long-awaited fountain-of-youth treatment for aging, weak, wrinkled facial skin? Frankly, it is not a miracle, but it is a help. It does not take the place of a face lift or chemical peel. It is also not capable of taking a very wrinkled face and making it look young again. It is more appropriate to think of retinoic acid as a medicine that, if used very faithfully for a long time, may *slow or decelerate* the "aging process." If it does that for you, it is enough. If it slowly rebuilds collagen support tissue in the dermis, makes some wrinkles less apparent, smooths skin tone, stops precancerous lesions, and gives facial skin a brighter look, it is certainly worthwhile.

Guidelines for use. Retinoic acid can cause redness, peeling, and itching if not used cautiously and carefully. Most individuals have some problems with this medication but can tolerate it and benefit from it if properly instructed. Individuals who wish to use retinoic acid are *strongly urged* to consult a dermatologist for guidance. In general, the rules for retinoic acid use are these:

1. *Start with a diluted medication.* A way to accomplish this is to dilute Retin A .05 percent cream with any light moisturizing lotion or cream. You can put a pea-sized dab of Retin A cream in your palm, add an equal amount of moisturizing cream, and thoroughly mix it with your finger. An alternative is to squeeze out an entire tube of Retin A into a small jar and thoroughly mix in an equal portion of moisturizing cream.

2. *Use very sparingly.* A quarter of a teaspoon is *plenty* to cover a face. Use less than that if you can.

3. *Begin treatment* no more often than every other evening. Leave retinoic acid cream on overnight. The nights you are not using retinoic acid cream, use a moisturizer.

4. *Be careful of eyelids.* Eyelid skin is very sensitive and will just not tolerate retinoic acid.

5. *Redness and peeling may occur.* If it is only a little, just put up with it. If it is a lot, stop using retinoic cream on those sensitive areas for a few days, then start again, perhaps more carefully.

6. *Persevere.* Skin becomes more tolerant to retinoic acid as it is used, so be persistent. Many individuals have difficulty with this medicine in the beginning, but find they can use it more often and in more concentrated form as time goes by.

7. *Always use a sunblocking lotion* in the morning. A creamy type that does not contain PABA is the best choice. Try Solbar P.F. (PABA-Free) creamy type. Individuals with very oily skin should use Solbar P.F. oil-free liquid type.

If you are interested in using retinoic acid, plan on using this medicine regularly—daily if you can—for a year, then less often for as long as you want to look your best. Be sure to use a good sunblocking product on your face every day, for only when sun damage is prevented can retinoic acid do enough for you to make the difference you want.

Alpha-Hydroxy Acids ("Fruit Acids," Lactic and Glycolic Acids and Others in This Family)

These substances may help "rejuvenate" skin to some degree. Alpha-hydroxy acids are usually added to moisturizing products. At least two products in this group are now marketed; they are listed in chapter 11.

For years dermatologists used these substances in moisturizing creams to treat extremely dry, flaky skin. They are generally more effective for this purpose than are regular moisturizers. There is recent interest in the effect of these substances in erasing wrinkles. Short-term studies have shown improvement in wrinkling; it is not now known if any long-term benefit will be gained from the use of alpha-hydroxy acids.

The way these substances work is by removing dry, dead surface cell plates, thus leaving the stratum corneum layer thinner, brighter, and more supple (less crinkly). At the time of this writing, it has *not* been shown that beneficial effects also occur in the dermis.

The drawback to the use of these substances is that on many faces they cause stinging and irritation—sometimes lots of it. The products available now may be more appropriate for dry hands and legs than for wrinkled faces.

Ascorbic Acid

Ascorbic acid is vitamin C, and it is essential to the skin's production of collagen (the substance critical to the skin's strength, thickness, and resilience). Recent evidence indicates that in older age we do become deficient in vitamin C. This deficiency may play a role in the skin thinning and wrinkling in older age.

So taking vitamin C supplements daily may improve aged skin, or at least help prevent age-related changes in skin. That's only a maybe. It hasn't been proven, but it may help some. Taking vitamin C daily seems a safe enough practice, and 500 milligrams daily is probably enough.

What about putting ascorbic acid (vitamin C) in a skin-care cream and "feeding" the skin's collagen-making ability? That may help too, but at the time of this writing we don't really know. Much more research needs to be done on the formulation of products in which ascorbic acid is stable (doesn't break down) and which encourage the penetration of ascorbic into the dermis, where it is needed. Remember, not much of what we put on the skin's surface actually penetrates past the thin top skin layer.

At the time of this writing we know of only one good ascorbic acid product that is being marketed: Avon Collagen Booster.

SUN DAMAGE
SUN PROTECTION

QUESTION:
> If I tan easily and deeply, am I safe sunbathing or going to a tanning salon?

ANSWER:
> A suntan does offer some protection against sun damage. Excessive sun exposure can still cause problems: wrinkles, skin cancers, and other *permanent* skin changes. Tanning parlors advertise that they are "safer" than sunlight. That is generally true when it comes to skin cancer. It is *not* true when it comes to skin "aging," for the rays emitted by such artificial sources may be more deeply damaging to skin than natural sunlight.

If you're like most, you have a love-hate relationship with the sun. You *love* what the sun can do for the color of your skin. And it is true that most of us look better a little tanned. It is also true that sunning seems to impart a feeling of well-being and vigor.

But you're going to *hate* the damage the sun is doing to your skin, which will show up years later. Tanned skin *is* damaged skin—the release of pigment into the skin (basically, what a tan is) is the body's response to prevent further damage. The response is slow—it takes several days to build up melanin—but the real damage (which won't show up for years) starts with the first exposure. In fact, most of what is called "aging" is actually photoaging, or damage done by the sun. Tanned skin gets old before its time. The sunlight that stimulates this browning causes more cell damage than the tan may prevent.

Exposure to the sun's ultraviolet (UV) radiation is more harmful to facial skin than biological aging, dryness, habits like smoking and drinking, or lack of proper skin care.

TAN NOW, PAY LATER

The problem with sun damage is that it isn't visible right away. It appears five to twenty years down the road. That time lag is deceptive—you may think you're getting off scot-free because your skin looks great now. In fact, a little tan is an incentive to get tanner. And this exposure will surface in the form of wrinkles, pebbly skin texture, uneven pigmentation, lines, age spots, liver spots, skin cancer (including malignant melanoma), and precancerous lesions.

These are forever—they don't fade with your tan. Not a pretty picture. But there's another cost to sun exposure: dollars spent on cosmetic and skin-care and -repair products, and on plastic surgeons and dermatologists.

Save yourself time, money, and worry—invest in a good sunscreen product (see guidelines on page 56) and apply it religiously every single day, no matter what the season. The money you spend on a sunscreen now may save you the $1,500 to $8,000 (American Society of Plastic and Reconstructive Surgeon guidelines) it costs for a face lift to redrape sagging, wrinkled, sun-damaged skin. It may save you the costs and scars of skin cancer surgery. It could even save your life, for we know now that sunburning fair skin is the leading cause of the deadly skin cancer malignant melanoma.

WHO GETS SUN DAMAGE?

Everyone, whether you tan or burn. Of course, fair-skinned, light-haired, light-eyed individuals are harmed far more by ultraviolet light exposure than are those with darker skin, hair, and eyes. Those who tan easily and well suffer less sun damage than those who do not, but they still suffer damage.

WHEN DOES SUN DAMAGE OCCUR?

• Sun damage is intentionally inflicted each time sunbathing, in natural or artificial light, is done.
• Sun damage is accidentally inflicted each time the face is exposed to the sun. The few short minutes spent walking to the car, running to the deli to pick up lunch, shopping, going out to get the mail, add up to hours of facial sun exposure. It is as important to protect the face from this kind of incidental sun exposure as it is to avoid intentional exposure.
• Sun damage can occur even on overcast days. Clouds, which consist of water droplets, transmit nearly 60 percent of the sun's radiation.

• Sun damage can also occur in the winter. Just because it isn't summer doesn't mean you're not getting solar exposure. Watch out for snow and ice, which reflect 90 percent of the sun's rays.

• Sun damage can occur underwater. UV light penetrates up to three feet below the surface of the water, and water droplets themselves act as magnifying glasses, intensifying the sun's effects.

• Sun damage can occur under an umbrella or visor. Sand, water, and concrete reflect sun up and under such shades.

• Sun damage can occur in any type of tanning parlor, even in those advertised as safe.

SHEDDING LIGHT ON THE RAYS

Sunlight is a mixture of both long-wavelength ultraviolet (UV) light (so-called UV-A rays) and midwavelength UV light (UV-B rays). Until recently, UV-A rays were dubbed "tanning rays," while UV-B rays were known as "burning rays." UV-A rays were considered "safe" rays, but this is no longer the case. While they account for most of the tanning effect of ultraviolet light, it is possible to get quite a burn from UV-A. It just takes longer. UV-A does penetrate the skin quite deeply and is primarily responsible for damage to the dermis, in the form of wrinkles. Since UV-A radiation is far more plentiful than UV-B radiation at any given time and damages the skin's support system, you can see why it is no longer considered harmless—and why tanning parlors, which use bulbs that produce mostly UV-A light are especially dangerous to the future condition of your skin.

UV-B rays do not penetrate skin very deeply. They are primarily responsible for sunburning and skin cancer formation. They produce some tanning and also cause damage to the dermis.

There is overlap in the effects of these two kinds of ultraviolet light. Both A and B rays cause tanning and burning—it just takes longer to burn with UV-A. UV-A rays also augment the damage potential of UV-B rays. Double trouble! And both cause damage to facial skin. Don't let anyone tell you otherwise.

As if these two factors weren't enough, new studies implicate another type of light—infrared, which is basically heat—in skin damage. Although it is unclear how much damage infrared light can do, it is thought to augment the damage done by ultraviolet light.

The Effects of Ultraviolet Light on Facial Skin

When sunlight strikes skin, many complex changes occur. In the epidermal layer, melanocyctes in the epidermis produce melanin pigment—that's what causes tanning; epidermal cells are altered, which may produce skin cancers and sunburns; and stratum corneum cells thicken, in an effort to physically block further ultraviolet penetration. In the deeper, dermis layer, ultraviolet light, especially the longer-wavelength rays, pass through the epidermis into the dermis and hurt it badly. These rays affect the foundation of the skin, thinning and weakening the collagen understructure. When the basement of the skin starts to crumble, skin at the surface sags into wrinkles and lines.

SUN PROTECTION

Always protect your skin from the sun. Start young and continue it henceforth if you want your facial skin to be as beautiful as it can be for as long as possible. Sun damage starts in childhood and continues throughout life. Every little bit of new damage adds up. Studies show that it takes only one severe burn in childhood to double the risk of getting skin cancer. And since most effects of sun damage (except sunburn) take years to show up, most individuals do not realize the amount of sun damage they have sustained until it is too late.

And what if you have been a sun worshipper most of your life? It's never too late to start protecting your skin. Skin does repair sun damage, but extremely slowly. You can't expect miracles, but you can expect some slowing of the sun-aging clock. Follow these guidelines to protect your skin from the sun:

Avoid all facial sun exposure. This is an absolute rule for the fair. The darker-complected can bend this rule, but not to the breaking point. Along the same line, it makes sense to avoid tanning parlors and the use of a sun reflector or a sunlamp.

Wear a wide-brimmed hat when outdoors. A hat can block some of the direct impact of solar radiation. Choose a tightly woven straw or cloth hat; if you can see through it, ultraviolet light can get through to your skin. Beware of the bounce-back effect from reflective surfaces such as sand, water, and concrete. Don't forget to apply sunscreen to your face even when you wear a sunhat.

Use sunblocking products. These are probably your best defense against sun damage. The products currently available are very good, though not yet perfect.

Sunblocking products are rated and labeled with a sun protection factor (SPF) number that gives the consumer an approximate indication of how effective the product is. The numbers usually range from

2 to 15, although some of the newer products claim SPF values all the way up to 50. The higher the number, the more protection the product gives.

SPF is an indication of how much time you can safely spend in the sun without suffering a burn if you use the product. For example, if your bare skin would normally burn in 10 minutes, the use of a product with an SPF of 15 would allow you to spend 150 minutes (10 × 15 = 150), or two and a half hours, in the sun without burning the skin.

It is possible to tan with a sunscreen. The lower the SPF, the greater the amount of UV rays that reach your skin. The formula for light transmittance is one over the SPF number. A product with an SPF of 2 allows ½ of the UV radiation to reach your skin; an SPF of 15, $\frac{1}{15}$ of the UV. But remember, a little tan is a little sun damage; a deeper tan is more sun damage.

It is always better to use a product with a higher SPF number than you think you need. SPF numbers are generated under laboratory conditions, so they don't take into account such real-world factors as wind, perspiration, and friction—all of which can lower the effectiveness of the product. Even the way you apply it (most of us tend to use less than we should and slap it on rather than studiously applying it) affects how much protection your skin gets from a product. Under such conditions, an SPF 10 may really give only the protection of an SPF 8. That's a persuasive argument for using the new superhigh-SPF products—using an SPF 30 under real-life conditions may give you the SPF 15 that you're counting on.

Although the SPF rating allows you to extend your time in the sun, it is important to realize that once you've used up that exposure time, reapplying a sunscreen *will not extend it.* If you use a sunscreen to enjoy two and a half hours of burn-free sun exposure, a second application of the product after the first two and a half hours will not protect for another two and a half hours in the sun.

Wear makeup. Makeup seems like a fine and very cosmetically acceptable way to protect skin from incidental sun exposure. It is—to a degree. Lipstick acts as a physical barrier to the sun; that may be why more men than women get lip cancer. The powder forms (not the cream formulations) of ordinary makeup—loose powders, eye shadows, foundations—seem to scatter light off and away from the skin surface. But it's better not to count on these as a sole source of sun protection.

Some foundations contain sunscreens, but there is just one little catch: Very few of them are labeled with an SPF, so you cannot judge the degree of protection this "contains-sunscreen" product affords. Since you now know that you should be using something with an SPF number of 15 or higher, you just cannot trust foundations that are not labeled with that number. What you can do is apply a sunscreen to your face before you apply your foundation.

THE CHEMISTRY OF SUNSCREENS

Sunscreens contain certain active ingredients that absorb UV radiation. And they do a pretty good, though not a perfect, job. Some chemicals that block UV-B don't absorb UV-A, and some that block UV-A let in UV-B. With the increasing evidence that UV-A is as bad for skin as UV-B, paying close attention to ingredients is even more important.

What you want is a "full-spectrum" sunscreen—one that contains ingredients that block both UV-A and UV-B. In general, sunscreens with an SPF of 15 or higher contain both UV-A and UV-B blockers, while those with an SPF below 15 contain UV-B blockers only.

Here are the most-used sunscreen chemicals:

UV-B blockers. PABA, or para-aminobenzoic acid, is the original compound that made "invisible" sunscreens possible. Prior to this, sunscreens were opaque sunblocks—mostly that white zinc oxide paste—that physically blocked the sun's rays. PABA was good, but the second-generation PABA esters (padimate-O, padimate-A, octyl dimethyl PABA) are better. PABA stains clothing yellow (especially cotton and linen) and can cause stinging and allergic reactions, while PABA esters cause less staining and fewer reactions than pure PABA.

Cinnamates are also B blockers but are more easily washed off than PABA—not a great choice if you perspire heavily or swim.

UV-A blockers. Benzophenones (oxybenzone, sulisobenzone, methoxybenzone) are not the greatest UV-B blockers, but are effective absorbers of UV-A.

Anthranilates (menthyl and homomenthyl-N-acetyl) are moderately effective in absorbing UV-A and UV-B.

Salicylates (homomenthyl salicylate) absorb UV-A.

SUNSCREEN SENSITIVITY

For all their good skin-saving properties, sunscreens can also cause some skin reactions, especially on sensitive facial skin. These include burning, stinging, redness, and itching—even breakouts. You may experience a reaction due to contact with the active ingredient itself—a contact dermatitis—or due to a combination of ultraviolet exposure and the active ingredient—a photocontact dermatitis. This doesn't mean you should give up using sunscreens. It simply means that you should switch sunscreens. Be sure that you aren't applying sunscreen to already irritated or sunburned skin—it will surely sting. What causes sunscreen allergic reactions:

PABA and its chemical relatives, padimate-O, padimate-A, and octyldimethyl PABA are the main culprits in sunscreen allergic reactions and/or just plain stinging and irritation. PABA is much worse in this department than its chemical relatives. The increasing use of sunscreens that contain these ingredients seems to be paralleled by an increasing incidence of reactions to them. As many as 20 percent of sunscreen users have become either allergic to these chemicals or at least intolerant of facial use of them.

For these reasons, we recommend PABA-free sunscreens for facial use. If you tolerate the facial use of sunscreens containing PABA or its relatives, then it's fine for you to use them. But any sign of stinging or irritation should signal you to change to a PABA-free product. Such products are usually labeled "PABA-free." If not, just read the ingredients list on the package.

Alcohol, found in alcohol-based sunscreens (usually those labeled for oily skin), can sting or irritate dry or sensitive skin. If you have hay fever or asthma, you may have especially dry, sensitive (atopic) skin. Try a lotion- or cream-based product.

Fragrances and preservatives may also trouble skin, so watch for any that may have troubled you in the past.

Patch Testing

To avoid learning the hard way which sunscreen is the wrong one for you, do a patch test before buying a sunscreen. Take a sample from a store tester, apply it to a small patch of skin on the inner elbow, and cover with a Band-Aid. After twenty-four hours, remove the Band-Aid and expose the area to fifteen minutes of sunlight. If you are sensitive to the product, a reaction—redness, swelling—will appear in this area the next day.

WAYS TO TURN A SUNSCREEN INTO A FACE SAVER

• Apply it daily. Tape a reminder to your bathroom or makeup mirror until using sunscreen becomes as automatic as brushing your teeth or combing your hair.

• Use an SPF 15 product all year round, or at the very least from April to October, when the sun is strongest.

• Apply sunscreen at least twenty minutes before exposing your face to the sun, in order to allow penetration into the stratum corneum, giving the skin better protection.

• If you have dry to normal skin, smooth on a sunscreen instead of a moisturizer under your foundation. That way, you won't forget to put it on.

• Application tip for real scorcher days: Apply sunscreen in cool conditions—in an air-conditioned room or a cool bathroom. The product may not apply evenly on skin slippery with perspiration. Also, perspiration (like any form of water) washes away sunscreen protection.

• If the alcohol-based sunscreen you use for your oily skin stings, you're applying it too late. Apply well before skin gets sweaty. If it stings when it gets into your eyes, next time circle both eyes with a sunscreen stick. The waxes in this product not only make it stay put but keep out other stinging sunscreens.

• Apply any sunscreen product generously. Skimping lowers the SPF protection.

RECOMMENDED SUNSCREENS

PABA-FREE AND PABA-ESTER PRODUCTS
Drugstore Products
PreSun 29 Sensitive Skin Sunscreen
Neutrogena Sunscreen (SPF 15)
T/I Pharmaceuticals TiScreen Lotion (SPF 15+)
Person & Covey Solbar P.F. Lotion
Greitzer Piz Buin Exclusit Extreme (SPF 15)
Coppertone Waterbabies Sunblock Lotion (SPF 15) and Sunblock P.F. Liquid Cream
    (SPF 25)
Total Eclipse PABA-free Sunblock Lotion (SPF 15)

Department Store Products
Avon Sun Seekers Ultra Sunsafe Sunblocking Lotion (SPF 15)
Clarins Total Sunscreen (SPF 18)

PABA-CONTAINING PRODUCTS FOR DRY SKIN
Drugstore Products

Westwood Presun Facial Sunscreen (SPF 15)
Nivea Moisturizing Sun Block Lotion (SPF 15 and 25)
Johnson & Johnson Sunblock Lotion (SPF 20)
Johnson & Johnson Sunblock Cream (SPF 24)
Schering Plough Super Shade 15 or 25

Department Store Products

Sebastian Ultrablock (SPF 29)
Estée Lauder Super Sun Block (SPF 20)
Clinique Face Zone Sun Block (SPF 15)
Elizabeth Arden Superblock Cream 34

PABA-CONTAINING PRODUCTS FOR OILY SKIN
Drugstore Products

Carter Sea & Ski Block Out Sunblock Cream Lotion (SPF 30)
Westwood PreSun 15
Eclipse Oil Free (SPF 15)
Solbar SPF 15

Department Store Products

Biotherm Oil Free Sun Protector (SPF 15)
Clinique Oil Free Sun Block SPF 15 (nonstaining formula)
Chanel Sun Shelter Cream Haute Protection (SPF 15)
Elizabeth Arden SunScience Oil Free Ultra Block (SPF 15)
Elizabeth Arden Oil Free Tanning Gel (SPF 15)

SUNSCREENS IN STICK FORM
Drugstore Products

Johnson & Johnson Sunblock Stick (SPF 20)
Total Eclipse Lip and Face Sunscreen Protectorant (SPF 15)
Presun 15 Sunscreen Stick
Bonne Bell Weatherproofer

Department Store Products

Chanel Protection Extreme Sun Shelter Face Block

SUNBLOCKING PRODUCTS
Drugstore Products

Manhattan Ice Le Zinc (zinc oxide in bright yellow, orange, pink, and blue)
Schering-Plough Coppertone Zinka Ztick (colorful zinc oxide)

Department Store Products

Clinique Continuous Coverage
Estée Lauder Total Sun Block Creme (SPF 23)

THE BEST, SAFEST TAN OF ALL—FAKING IT

The various tan-in-a-bottle products work best on small areas, like the face. With these skin-preparation/application tips, you can get natural-looking color without unnecessary UV exposure. Here's how to put on a sunny face:

• *Product options.* Makeup-type bronzers, available in lotion, powder, and gel form, for an hours-long tan; self-tanning lotions or creams, for a two- or four-day tan.

• *Skin-preparation tips.* Exfoliate skin with a loofah or scrubbing product (see suggestions in chapter 10). The smoother your skin, the more evenly you can apply a "tan." Apply the product only to clean, well-dried skin—this also affects how the color is absorbed by stratum corneum.

• *Application specifics for liquid bronzing makeups.* Pour a quarter-size amount onto a cosmetic sponge—slightly damp for lotion, dry for creams and gels. Smooth on, using long strokes—don't dot, as this will cause streaks. Creams and lotions, also known as "sport tints," are basically light foundation-type products; gels are sheer and "tan" skin transparently. Remove them by regular facial washing.

• *Application specifics for bronzing powders.* Smooth on with a powder puff, using long, light strokes. Don't rub powder into skin. Smooth away excess with a brush. Use powders selectively: on cheekbones, bridge of nose, chin—just where the sun would hit your face. Remove it with regular facial washing.

• *Application specifics for self-tanning lotions and creams.* Smooth on one thin coat; follow it fifteen minutes later with a more generous layer, to prevent streaking and missed spots. Self-tanners contain a chemical (most commonly DHA, dihydroxyacetone) that stains the stratum corneum in about three hours. The color gradually fades as the stratum corneum is sloughed off. A self-tanner can be used several times during a day to get a darker color. It is not the same as a tan accelerator, which is advertised to promote faster tanning when you go out in the sun. Color-test a self-tanner before applying it, to see how your skin takes the shade. You may have better luck with another product.

Remember, with any of these products you have a fake tan—and that means no protection from the sun. If you want to go outside sporting your fake tan, put on a sunscreen, *under* the bronzing makeup or *over* the self-tanner.

RECOMMENDED SELF-TANNING PRODUCTS

BRONZING LOTIONS AND CREAMS
Lancôme Bienfait du Matin
Charles of the Ritz Perfect Protection Makeup

BRONZING GELS
Bonne Bell Bronzing Gel
Bain de Soleil's Le Bronze Sheer Suncolor

BRONZING POWDERS
Clinique Think Bronze Transparent Buffer
Guerlain Terracotta Bronzing Powder
Revlon Pure Radiance Pressed Powder, "Original Sunglow"

SELF-TANNERS
Estée Lauder Self-Sun Action Tanning Creme
Germaine Monteil Soleil Self-Tanning Creme
Biotherm Self Tanning Lotion
Prescriptives Sun-Free Tanner

9

DAILY CLEANSING
The Simple, Inexpensive Way

QUESTION:
> I just bought a very expensive "deep cleanser" that seems heavy and greasy. Will this help unclog my pores?

ANSWER:
> Most products in this category are no better than inexpensive cold cream and may actually clog pores rather than unclog them. If you want your skin clean, always use a *lathering* cleansing product after you have used the heavy, greasy one. By the way, no cleansers are really "deep" cleansing.

Cleansing is indeed important for beautiful, healthy skin. But cleansing need not be complicated or expensive; simple routines and inexpensive products are as good.

Good cleansing is especially important and helpful in oily skin types, where pores tend to be large, the buildup of surface cells can make the skin look dull, and problems like acne breakouts and seborrheic dermatitis often occur. Good cleansing really improves the look and texture of oily skin and helps prevent those problems.

Cleansing is also important for the more delicate and trouble-free skin types, but not nearly so important as it is for the oilier skin types.

So facial skin cleansing really must be individualized. You can easily learn to develop your own simple program to suit *your* skin. You know something about your skin type from reading previous chapters. Now read about *cleansing* and put all this together into a routine that fits your own skin.

Skin-cleansing product advertising no doubt has you confused. Every cosmetic company has its cleansing products, which you are told are the best. There are products that claim to be "deep cleansing," or "exfoliative," or extra gentle, extra thorough, etc. Some lines have elaborate regimens that they recommend you follow. There is indeed much available to spend your money on when it comes to cleansing your face!

Good cleansing removes dirt, microbes, skin oils, dead stratum corneum cells, and all cosmetic products from the surface of the skin.

It is a fact that many cleansing products and routines do not cleanse well. It is *generally* true that cleansing products that are lathering and water-rinsable clean skin far better than those that are not.

TYPES OF SKIN CLEANSERS

Do not be confused by the many products and programs offered at cosmetic counters and in advertisements. Cleansing agents fall into a few simple categories. Here is help in understanding cleansing products.

Cleansing Creams, Lotions, and Milks

"Tissue-off" types. These products are applied to the skin, massaged in a little, and removed with tissues. They leave a residue of skin oils, dirt, microbes, makeup, *and the cleanser itself!*

They are useful for removing heavy oil-based makeup, masking cream, stage makeup, and waterproof makeup, but by themselves they do *not* clean well. If cleansers of this type are used, they must be followed by a thorough washing with a lathering cleanser (see below). It is interesting that most of the really expensive facial skin-cleansing products fall into this category. It is also interesting that plain old inexpensive cold cream is as good as any of them. Basically, that's all these so-called cleansing creams are—variations of the cold cream formula with a few extra ingredients mixed in. Cleansing lotions have the same basic formulation with extra water to make them more liquid. This translates as less pull on skin and somewhat easier removal than with a cream, but these too should be followed up by a lathering cleanser for thorough removal.

Skin-type recommendations. Tissue-off cleansers are best suited for removing makeup (especially waterproof) from dry, average, and delicate skin. They may be too oily for oily or acne-prone skin, and failure to remove such cleansers completely often leads to problems—blocked pores, large pores, blackheads, whiteheads, acne, seborrheic dermatitis, dull-looking skin.

TISSUE-OFF CLEANSERS
Drugstore Products
Pond's Essential Cleansing Lotion
Dorothy Gray Magic Moisturizing Cleansing Lotion
Jergens All Purpose Face Cream

Department Store Products
Orlane Ligne Active Lait Demaquillant
Germaine Monteil Super Moist Cleansing Lotion
Lancôme Galatee Milky Creme Cleanser

Water-rinse-off types. These cleansers are applied to the skin, massaged in, and rinsed away with water. Provided that they really rinse off easily and completely (some of the best ones even lather a little), they are good cleansers. They usually remove makeup well—all but the heaviest, oiliest foundations. Foundations that are not easily removed by cleansers of this type probably are too heavy to use at all.

Skin-type recommendations. Those with delicate, sensitive, or nonoily skin can use these with no problem. Those with average to oily skin can use them too, provided use is followed by a lathering cleanser for a double cleansing effect.

Those with skin somewhere in between can also use a cleansing cream at night and a lathering cleanser in the morning to get the benefits of both systems.

RINSE-OFF CLEANSERS
Drugstore Products
Doak Pharmaceutical Formula 405 Facial Skin Cleansing Lotion
Almay Oil Control Facial Cleanser
Aquanil Lotion
Cetaphil Lotion

Department Store Products
Lancôme Douceur Demaquillante Nutrix
Clinique Extremely Gentle Cleansing Cream
Prescriptives Essential Cleansing Gel
Controle De Lancôme Priming Cleanser for Oily Skin

Lathering Cleansers

Lathering cleansing agents are the most important category, for they simply clean the best. They should be part of almost everyone's cleansing routine. They are the *only* cleansing product that most skins really need, because they adhere to and dissolve what we are trying to cleanse off skin. Then, with the water rinse, they foam and literally float the dissolved impurities, oils, makeup, microbes, and dead skin cells down the drain.

Lathering cleansers come in many forms—soap and nonsoap, liquid and bar. There's a lathering cleanser to suit any skin, from the oiliest to the most delicate.

Plain soap. This soap is the prototype of lathering cleansers. Since the time when melted lard was first mixed with lye to make the sudsing stuff, many changes have occurred in what we still call soap. Many of the modern lathering cleanses are not soap, technically speaking, but have the same effect.

Most true soaps are slightly alkaline (high pH), so the natural pH of skin (5.5 to 6.5) is temporarily altered by washing, but it is restored quickly—sometimes within minutes, as oil glands continue their output. Soaps are available in bar and liquid form, which is the same formulation with extra water added.

Skin-type recommendations. There's a soap for nearly every skin type. In general, you can't go wrong by choosing and using a "mild" soap.

PLAIN SOAPS
Drugstore Products
Ivory Soap
Purpose Soap
Neutrogena (various formulas for different skin types)

Superfatted soaps. These soaps contain extra fat—usually lanolin, olive oil, or cocoa butter. The higher the fat content of a soap, the less drying it is. Extra fat makes the lather less alkaline, so less oil is removed from the face. The soap's complement of extra fat means that some is probably left on the skin surface, contributing to the less dry—less tight feeling after use.

Skin-type recommendations. Superfatted soaps are fine for those with dry to normal skin, but those with oily or acne-prone skin should steer clear to keep clear.

SUPERFATTED SOAPS
Drugstore Products
Basis Soap
Neutrogena for Dry Skin
Steifel Oilatum
Beiersdorf Eucerin

Transparent soaps. Transparent soaps may have a higher fat content than superfatted soaps, and they also contain glycerine and alcohol (part of what makes them transparent). One drawback to these soaps is that they dissolve rapidly, both through routine use and through sitting in a wet soap dish. Make your bar last longer by patting it dry after each use and making sure there's no residual water in the soap dish.

Skin-type recommendations. Best for normal to dry skin, delicate or sensitive skin.

TRANSPARENT SOAPS
Drugstore Products
Neutrogena (formulas for dry skin, oily skin, acne-prone skin)
Pears Transparent Soap
Jergens Clear Complexion Bar

Milled soaps. The milling process compresses soap solids to squeeze out air and water. Due to this concentration, the resulting bar has a higher fat content than unmilled soaps. These bars are more expensive than unmilled soaps, but do last longer. How to tell if your soap is milled? If it floats, it's not; since they contain no air pockets, milled soaps sink.

Skin-type recommendations. These soaps are good for all skin types as they are specifically formulated for different complexion needs. Use the one formulated for your skin type.

MILLED SOAPS
Department Store Products
Clinique Facial Soap
Erno Lazlo Hydraphel Cleansing Treatment
Discipline Skin Care The Only Soap
Prescriptives Essential Cleansing Bar

Soapless soaps. These are known in the cosmetic industry as "syndets," because they are synthetic soaps that contain detergents, usually petroleum derivatives, instead of animal or vegetable fats. Most modern soaps, whether liquid or bar, are syndets. These are less alkaline than basic soap. Many are labeled "pH-balanced." Label clues: The product is called a "beauty bar" or "bath bar," or lauryl sulfate appears up near the top of the ingredients list.

Skin-type recommendations. They rinse off quickly and easily and are good for sensitive skins. If you live in a hard-water area, a syndet is a good choice because it leaves little residue.

SYNDETS
Drugstore Products
Westwood Lowila Cake
pHresh 3.5 (liquid)
Cooper Aveeno (bar)
Lever Bros. Dove
Neutrogena Liquid Facial Cleansing Formula
Bonne Bell Ten-O-Six Cleansing Bar

Department Store Products
Esteem Thorough Cleansing Bar

TEN-SECOND RINSE TEST

All this talk about how cleansers rinse off the skin may have you confused. Why should you care about how a cleanser rinses? Well, the more easily it rinses, the less residue is left on the skin and the "milder" or "gentler" a cleanser is considered. Residue left on the skin is a potential source of irritation. How can you tell how your cleanser rinses? Wash your hands with the cleanser you usually use. Rinse and then run your index finger down a mirror. If your finger leaves a streak, that's residue and your cleanser doesn't rinse well. (Or your rinse technique leaves something to be desired!) Now rub your fingers together—does the skin feel slick, slippery, greasy? That's cleanser residue.

EYE MAKEUP REMOVERS

Taking off eye makeup with a cleanser is problematic—most sting or irritate eyes. The solution? A separate prewashing step to take off makeup. There are many special products—in liquid, gel, or pre-soaked-pad forms—sold for this purpose, and they are especially useful in removing waterproof eye makeup, which does not come off with water.

Warning: Eyelid skin is the thinnest and most sensitive skin on the face and is very easily irritated by cleansing products and overvigorous cleansing motions (wiping, rubbing, etc). If you experience dermatitis—redness, itching, rash—on the eyelids, one of your first suspects should be the makeup remover.

EYE MAKEUP REMOVERS AND CONTACT LENS WEARERS

If you wear contact lenses, always remove them before taking off eye makeup. Eye makeup removers contain oils or solvents that can seep into eyes, clouding and staining lenses as well as attracting further deposits. If you wear extended-wear lenses, use a remover formulated for lens wearers. These are oil-free. Extended-wear lenses in particular have a high water content that makes them especialy vulnerable to staining and clouding.

In general, eye makeup removal should be followed by a lathering cleanser to remove all traces of remover and makeup. Be sure to rinse the eye area thoroughly with plain water after using a makeup remover, to wash away all traces of the product. Some simple, inexpensive, and practically trouble-free eye-area cleansers are cold cream and mineral oil. Gently massage one on and remove with a cotton ball. Follow this with a gentle lathering with baby shampoo, then rinse. Baby shampoo ("no more tears") won't irritate eyes. This technique works best with waterproof eye products.

Skin-type recommendations. Dry, sensitive skins do best with a product that contains oil, but an oily remover can stain clothing and pillowcases. Oil-free ones may be too harsh. Or go with cold cream or mineral oil as suggested. As for oily or acne-prone skin, oil-containing or oil-free products can be used—it's very rare to be oily or breakout-prone in the eye area. Just wash thoroughly after use.

EYE MAKEUP REMOVERS
Drugstore Products
Almay Non Oily Eye Makeup Remover (for lens wearers)
Pond's Cold Cream
Jergens All-Purpose Face Cream
Maybelline 100% Oil Free Eye Make-Up Remover
Aziza Eye Makeup Remover Pads
Johnson's Baby Oil
Revlon Special Eyes Micropure Eye Makeup Remover

Department Store Products
Clinique Oil Free Eye Makeup Remover
Lancôme Gentle Eye Makeup Remover Gel
Lancôme Effacil Gentle Eye Makeup Remover (contains thimerosal)
Laboratoire Pons Eye Care Remover (through eye-care specialists only)
Kelemata Eye Makeup Remover Lotion
Kelemata Eye Makeup Remover Pads

ASTRINGENTS, TONERS, AND FRESHENERS

These are used as the final step in many cleansing routines. If you wear makeup that "stains" or penetrates the stratum corneum slightly (instead of sitting on the skin surface), you'll find an astringent-type product helpful when it comes time to remove it.

In general, these products contain varying proportions of alcohol and water, plus color, fragrance, solvents (to dissolve and remove skin oil and stratum corneum cells), and moisturizer. Those labeled for oily skin (interchangeably known as fresheners and astringents) contain more and stronger solvents; those for dry or sensitive skin (known as clarifiers and toners), less.

They are fine to use if you like, but aren't needed if you have used a lathering cleanser correctly. They do make skin feel "fresher" and "cleaner"—usually the result of added methol or camphor, which evaporates when it comes into contact with the skin. And they seem to be satisfying for the "dirt" that appears on the cotton ball (really just more loose stratum corneum cells). It makes you feel you have gotten the very last bit of grime off your face. Note: They should never be used in the eye area or to remove eye makeup.

Skin-type recommendations. For oily skin with large pores, astringents do seem to make pores smaller temporarily . . . but so does soap. They are fine for normal skin. Some delicate faces may be irritated by these products—even those labeled "for dry or sensitive skin." Witch hazel, alcohol, zinc salts, and aluminum salts are all very drying. If irritation—redness, itching, extreme tightness that lasts several hours—erupts, don't use these. Don't feel you have to use one. As you've seen, your skin is plenty clean.

ASTRINGENTS, TONERS, AND FRESHENERS
Drugstore Products
Clairol Sea Breeze Antiseptic
Clairol Sea Breeze Antiseptic for Sensitive Skin
Dickinson's Witch Hazel
Almay Counter Balance Pore Lotion
Almay Moisture Balance Toner
Almay Moisture Renewal Toner
Almay Oil Control Toner
Allercreme Astringent for Oily Skin
Allercreme Skin Freshener

Department Store Products
Lancôme Tonique Douceur

Estée Lauder Mild Action Protection Tonic
Discipline Skin Care The Solution
Clinique Clarifying Lotion 1, 2, and 3

SIX WAYS TO CLEAN YOUR FACE BETTER

Does it seem too basic to tell you how to wash your face? Read these tips—you'll probably learn something new!

• *Start with clean tools.* Wash your hands before washing your face. No sense in "applying" additional dirt, bacteria, what-have-you to facial skin.

• *Turn on tepid water.* Hot water may feel more relaxing, seem more disinfecting, but it is more drying.

• *Don't overscrub.* You aren't going to get your skin any cleaner and you may end up irritating it. If you're pink hours after cleansing, you're scrubbing too hard—ease off. If you've got acne-prone skin, you may even cause a flare-up. Spare the elbow grease. You really don't need to rub your face to remove dirt, makeup, etc.—a gentle massaging action with the pads (the fleshy part) of your fingertips (or a washcloth, sponge, or brush) nudges away what you don't want on skin. Rule of thumb: The rougher the tool, the lighter your touch should be.

• *Rinse rapidly.* Don't let the cleanser sit on your skin and don't massage forever—you may force dirt, makeup, etc., into skin instead of cleaning it out!

• *Rinse thoroughly*—probably the most important and most overlooked step of all. Skin irritation—redness, dryness, stinging, tightness—may result from cleanser residue that wasn't rinsed away. What you should do: Rinse your face really well, until you think you've removed all traces of cleanser. Then rinse, rinse, rinse some more.

• *Rinse clean.* Your splashes after cleansing should be with clean water, not water that has been standing in the sink, full of dissolved cleanser and cleanser residue.

• *Pat dry.* Again, vigorous rubbing may feel good, but you should take it easy on facial skin.

CLEANSING TOOLS

Brushes, scrubbing pads, natural sea sponges, and washcloths are traditional cleansing tools.

Keep your tools clean! (That goes for fingertips, too.) Using the same washcloth time after time is not a good idea—it gets warm and wet and becomes a hospitable environment for bacteria. Change washcloths daily. One tip to get around having a full laundry hamper: Cut up an old bathtowel into small pieces to be used one at a time.

Cosmetic brushes should be rinsed thoroughly after each use. Shake well to remove excess water, and leave them to dry bristle side up. Brushes do wear out—figure on replacing yours once a year. Figure replacement costs in when you're pricing brushes—it can add up. In-store test for gentleness: Press bristles on your inner elbow. If it feels rough there, it'll feel rough on your face.

Natural sponges should be thoroughly rinsed, wrung, and left to air-dry. They should be replaced when they begin to break down and shred—about every nine months to a year. Synthetic sponges should be well rinsed and drained. Bacterial invasion is not such a problem with these—germs don't breed as readily in artificial fibers. These should be replaced when they don't rinse well. It's easy to overdo it with a synthetic sponge. There are ones formulated to be gentle (they're labeled that way), but even these should be used with lots of water and cleanser to protect the skin from abrasion.

Skin-type recommendations. They are especially useful for oily and nonsensitive faces, for they effectively remove dead skin cell buildup. Sensitive, easily irritated faces should not use cleansing brushes and sponges—a fingertip lathering is adequate for good cleansing of sensitive skin.

YOUR INDIVIDUAL CLEANSING ROUTINE

With some knowledge of cleansing products and how they work, and some understanding of your facial skin, you can create your own individual cleansing routine. Some hints:

Skin type. Any guidelines given are necessarily very general. Skin types vary so greatly that it is difficult to give a valid cleansing recipe for every one. Skin type is something to take into consideration when it comes to choosing products, but keep in mind that what counts is how the product performs on your skin, not what the label says.

Cleanser type. The best advice here is to choose the cleanser that feels best to you. That advice may sound simplistic, but it's really true. Note how your skin feels during and after product use. Do you like the feel of the cleanser on your skin? Other factors to take into consideration: the scent, the size, the shape, and above all the price of the product! And how can you tell if a cleanser is working for you? Zero in on your skin. Does it look and feel clean, healthy? Check your skin right after washing, then an hour or two later—does it still feel good? Does it feel soft and supple? Is it rash- and breakout-free? Some feeling of tightness or dryness after cleansing is normal. (If it is extreme, it means that the cleanser or the routine may be too harsh or that you have seborreheic dermatitis or a tendency to eczema.) Listen to feedback from others—comments that you look tired or look terrific can give you an idea of how the product works for you. When you're auditioning a new product, give it a week before you make any final decision. Of course, if you experience any signs of irritation, discontinue use immediately.

Do you need a skin-care regimen—soap, toner, moisturizer, mask, etc.? There are pluses and minuses to this approach. If you like what the cleanser in a certain line does for your skin, chances are you'll like the other products. The strength of a regimen is that all the products are keyed to your skin type and formulated to work together. When you mix and match from different lines, one product may cancel out another—you may use a mild soap for your dry skin and then top it off with a high-alcohol drying toner, for example. That doesn't mean you can't pull together your own assemblage of products from different lines that work for you. You just have to be more attentive. One more consideration: Don't feel you have to buy every product in the regimen—buy only the ones you'll use. What's the good of a product that just sits on the shelf?

Frequency. Twice daily is fine for most people. More often is seldom necessary unless you are very oily or really get dirty. Good cleansing before bedtime is essential to remove makeup and the day's dirt. If your skin feels tight or dry with two washings a day, use milder products and try to be more gentle with your skin.

The season of the year may determine not only how often you wash but what you use to wash. Hot, humid weather usually calls for more frequent and more thorough cleansing than is needed in cold, low-humidity wintertime.

Water type. Whether your tap water is hard or soft can have a bearing on your cleansing choices and routines. Calcium and magnesium levels are higher in hard water, and these can combine with regular soaps to leave a film on your skin. In this case, a syndet or other soapless cleanser is a smart move. How can you tell how hard or soft your water is? The easiest way is to run your hand around your tub or sink basin—if you feel a filmy residue or see a ring, you've got hard water. A call to your local health or water department can confirm the mineral concentration in your water.

In summary, there is really little mystery in skin cleansing. It is a simple, practical matter—much simpler and less mysterious than some cosmetic companies want you to think. The mystery to derma-tologists is the amount of time and money many individuals spend on cleansing. Some products and routines cost many times more than others that are just as good. Please, do not feel that somehow you are "cheating" your skin if you are unwilling or unable to spend big on cleansing products—it is just not necessary. Consider performance, not price, when it comes to cleansing.

SKIN TREATMENTS

10

QUESTION:
What will a "professional facial" do for me? How often should
I have one done?
ANSWER:
A professional facial feels great but isn't as important as you
might think.

In addition to the basic products for cleansing skin, there are a host of special treatments for occasional use, designed to supplement (and advertised to go one step further than) your daily cleansing. On the home-care front, you can choose from masks, scrubbing cleansers, and grains; you can even steam-clean your face. Professional facials are the prime offering of skin-care salons—backed up with a line of products and makeup for home care between treatments. Do you really need them? How much more cleansing does your skin really need? Can a salon facial cleanse skin any better than your at-home routine? Here's how to make some smart skin decisions on these treatments.

STEAMING FACIAL SKIN

One of the time-honoured rituals for cleansing skin is steaming. Since you now know that there is no such thing as "deep" cleansing, what does steaming really do? Steaming hydrates skin and softens the clumps of stratum corneum cells, and to some extent the upper portion of the waxy plugs of blackheads that sit in pores. Naturally, if steaming softens these plugs, making them easier to get up and out, that makes you think of removing blackheads with your fingers. Resist the temptation as much as you can—you're likely to make things worse, not better. The best follow-up to steaming is a mask or scrubbing cleanser—let it remove plugs. Any lesions still remaining should be left alone or examined by a dermatologist.

If you want to steam your face, do it right, please. It is easy to drift too close to too-hot vapors for too long. You can burn your skin with steam! The skin-safe way to steam at home: Simmer a pot of water on the range and remove it from the heat. Let it cool for a few minutes, until it's still hot but not at boiling temperature. Place the pot on a counter where you can lean over it, but get your face no closer than twelve inches from the water. Measure it with a ruler to be sure. To keep water vapor from dissipating into the air, "tent" a terrycloth towel over your head and the pot. You can toss a few herbs into the water, but these just make the steam smell nice and have no direct effect on your skin. If the steam is uncomfortable, stop and let the water cool a bit further.

A typical steaming session should last about five minutes—but not all at once. Lift your head once in a while. Longer steaming is not better, and should be avoided in the case of active acne or troubled skin—too much can provoke a breakout, much like summer's humidity.

SCRUB-TYPE CLEANSERS

These cleansers exfoliate, or scrub away, built-up layers of dead stratum corneum cells. This makes the skin look brighter and translucent. How, exactly? The natural process of shedding stratum corneum is not even—clumps of cells can accumulate. The result: When light hits the skin, it is not evenly reflected, so the skin looks dull. You can't feel this clumping effect, but you can see it—the skin looks grayish and dull. Any agent that removes accumulated cells and debris is in effect resurfacing the skin—uncovering the smooth, plumper layer of cells underneath—and making the skin look fresher and slightly glowing. This glow, of course, is temporary and due to increased local circulation.

Scrub cleansers consist of a lotion or creamy base with added abrasive material. Those for dry skin contain oil. Those for acne have a detergent base—polyexyethylene lauryl ether, for example. Some even contain salicylic acid, instead of or in addition to grains; it is a mild chemical exfoliant to lift away dead stratum corneum cells. They can also be purchased as dry grains you mix with water to form a paste.

The scrub cleansers that lather really do clean thoroughly. They are especially recommended for oily skin, which so often looks dull. Surface oil aids the clumping of surface cells by literally gluing them together. These cleansers may be used once weekly (or more often *if tolerated*); see the "Skin Treatment Schedule" on page 77.

Overuse will cause discomfort, stinging, chapping, scraped, abraded skin, and rashes. It is surprisingly easy to overdo it. Abraded skin not only feels bad, it is vulnerable to infection.

If you overdo it with a scrubber, pat the affected area clean with a clean washcloth and dab on some antibacterial ointment . . . and don't do it again! Discontinue scrubber use until the skin heals.

If you've adjusted the pressure and grains still seem to irritate your skin, try switching to a type with larger, rounded, or polyethylene grains. Some scrubbers, mostly the "natural"-grain type, contain jagged edged particles that can irritate skin. Or skip these altogether and try a mask if you want to treat your skin.

Getting the Best Results from a Scrubber

1. It's a good idea to wash (and steam, if you like) your face first instead of slapping on cleansing grains first thing. At the very least, hold a warm damp washcloth to your face for several seconds. Softening the skin first—with moisture or warmth—facilitates the exfoliating process.
2. To prevent abrasion, massage gently, using plenty of water to "buffer" the grainy portion of the cleanser.
3. Don't concentrate on any one area—you can't scrub out a blackhead the way you'd scrub out a stain from the sink.
4. Remove with water splashes, not a washcloth, which might be too much exfoliation.
5. Don't ever use grains or grainy cleansers on sunburned, windburned, or otherwise sensitive skin.
6. Follow up with a moisturizer suited to your skin. (See chapter 11.)

Do You Really Need a Scrubbing Product?

Can your skin benefit from using these scrubbers? While there are cosmetic benefits in exfoliating skin, just remember that you're doing the same thing when you bear down on a washcloth, lather up with a complexion brush, or use an abrasive sponge. Scrubbing cleansers seem to be a bit more efficient at this task and, properly used, may benefit your skin. An inexpensive alternative that works very well is cornmeal and water mixed to form a runny paste.

SCRUBBING CLEANSERS
Drugstore Products
Flori Roberts Derma Pure Facial
Stiefel Labs Brasivol Lathering Scrub Cleanser

Dorothy Gray Cleansing Grains
Clairol Sea Breeze Facial Scrub
Revlon Moon Drops Sluffing Masque
Coty Sweet Earth "Suds"

Department Store Products
Biotherm Gentle Facial Scrub
Clinique 7-Day Scrub Cream
Clinique Exfoliating Scrub
Estée Lauder Gentle Action Skin Polisher
Adrien Arpel Honey and Almond Scrub
Esteem Gentle Skin Sweeper
Prescriptives Skin Refiner and Skin Refining Gel
Lancôme Bienfait Demaquillant

MASKS

There are many mask (or masque) products available—cleansing, exfoliating, moisturizing, firming, revitalizing, and medicated. Unfortunately, there are as many claims for their skin effects—absorbing impurities, lifting away stubborn blackheads, deep cleansing, tightening pores, purifying skin, cleansing skin of pollutants.

What can they really do? Masks are quite good for brightening the look of the skin, because they remove some of the top layers of the stratum corneum and "pollutants"—dirt and makeup. Removing the irregular clumps of dead cells makes a smoother surface that reflects light better, thus giving a more refined, "newer" look and a smoother feel to skin. As for tightening pores, you should know better by now! Some masks make pores appear smaller, but this is only a temporary effect (in the neighborhood of two to three hours).

Skin does glow after you use a mask. This is another temporary effect, caused by local stimulation of the skin. As for the claim of erasing or easing facial lines, masks do seem to live up to that one. But how much of it is mask and how much the result of sitting quietly and relaxing is hard to tell. Again, this is a short-lived effect.

Basic Mask Types

Most cosmetic lines carry two types of masks—a cream-based formula to moisturize dry skin and one that contains clay to soak up excess oil from oily skin. Within that broad division, there are a few subcategories:

Harden-on-skin/rinse-off types. Mostly these are cleansing or exfoliating masks that are applied to the skin, left to dry for a while, and removed by rinsing. In general, a mask of this type is less abrasive than a scrubbing cleanser. If scrubbing cleansers irritate your skin, you may want to use only a mask. Most cleansing/exfoliating masks contain clay, fuller's earth, or kaolin, also known as China clay. Clay is mined from the earth and so is technically dirt, albeit a very refined and "clean" dirt. Some masks contain similarly refined mud. These seem to absorb some surface oil. Clay does absorb many times its weight in water. These ingredients work in concert with various other substances (for example, oatmeal) to create an abrasive effect.

Peel-off types. Some exfoliating masks and most "firming" masks are of this variety. Polyvinyl alcohol or vinyl acetate, both film-forming agents, give these masks their stretchy, plastic quality. These are left on the face to dry and are removed by peeling. As they dry, the mask latches on to loose stratum corneum cells. When it is peeled off, dead cells go with the mask.

As the mask dries on the skin, it causes a firming or tightening feeling, which is *strictly temporary*. This illusion of tightening and firming is nice but brief. Masks do not alter weak or sagging skin. The real benefit of most masks comes in removing them, rinsing or lifting away dead stratum corneum cells.

Soft/rinse-off types. So-called soft masks are either cream or gels. These are applied to skin, left on for a certain amount of time, and rinsed off. They do not dry on the skin and are better for on-the-dry-side skin. They often contain some sort of moisturizing ingredient. Do they really moisturize? To the degree that the mask itself forms a barrier between skin and environment, yes. However, the mask must come off at some point, and any protective or moisturizing effects are removed with it.

Soft masks are often tagged "refining" or "clarifying" and are designed to carry off any surface flaking via the rinsing, leaving skin smooth and brighter. Masks that claim to have refreshing or restorative effects ususally have a high water or alcohol content. As these evaporate, the skin feels fresher. Aromatic ingredients such as mint, menthol, or eucalyptus also contribute to the tingling, cooling effect.

Skin-type recommendations. Masks are fine to use occasionally when you feel like spending some time on yourself. Keep an eye on the time—don't let a mask sit on skin longer than the recommended time. That can overdry or irritate the skin. Normal to oily skin can handle the type that dries or peels away once or twice a week. The exfoliating types can be used once a week (or even more often) on

Skin-Treatment Schedule

Skin Types

	Normal	*Dry*	*Oily*	*Acne-Prone*	*Sensitive*
Mask Type and Timing	Mild/soothing 1X week	Moisturizing 2X month	Mud/clay Up to 2X weekly	Skip it	Mild gel or cream types 2X month
Scrubber Type and Timing	Grains, grainy scrub where needed (nose, chin) 1X weekly	Lotion or creamy types 1X weekly	Grainy scrubs Up to 2X weekly	Scrub on blackheads, whiteheads only 1X weekly	Avoid—may be too irritating
Steaming	Prescrub, mask use	Prescrub, mask use	Prescrub, mask use	Avoid—can cause flare-ups	Avoid—too irritating

oily skin. Delicate and sensitive skin should use masks with caution, for they may be irritating or drying. Once a week is not a hard and fast rule—you can use a mask once a month, for a special occasion, or seasonally—to "spring-clean" winter-dried skin, for example. See the "Skin Treatment Schedule" below for guidelines.

There are a few truly medicated masks that are useful in acne-prone skin. They are mentioned in chapter 14.

Can't match a mask to your skin type? You can also spot-apply masks, dabbing on clay- or mud-based ones in oily areas, others in not-so-oily areas—but be aware you'll be bearing double the cost, buying two masks instead of one. Better yet, dab a mask on problem areas of skin and let relatively problem-free skin just be.

MASKS FOR OILY SKIN
Drugstore Products
Chattem Labs Mudd Super Cleansing Treatment
Barbara Walden Mint Masque

Department Store Products
Adrien Arpel Sea-Mud Pack
Orlane Ligne Active Masque Bleu
Elizabeth Arden Velva Cream Mask
Christine Valmy Valmask I

MASKS FOR DRY SKIN
Drugstore Products
Revlon Moon Drops Honey Moisturizing Masque

Department Store Products
Biotherme Masque Net
Chanel Masque Creme Hydro-Protecteur/Active Moisture Supplement soft mask
Chanel Masque Lifting
Clarins Moisturizing Mask
Lancôme Masque No. 10
Orlane Ligne Integrale Masque Rose

SALON FACIALS

What can you realistically expect from a facial? Pampering, certainly, but noticeably cleaner or healthier skin? Only maybe.

Salons have entered the same high-tech age as cosmetics. You may be either impressed or intimidated by the array of machines and products devoted to skin cleansing, purifying, refreshing, rejuvenating, etc. Each salon has its own regimens and treatments for various skin types, but in general a facial includes the following:

- A skin analysis.
- Steaming—accomplished by a misting device that dispenses an even, warm (not hot) stream of vapor at the face.
- *Comedone extraction*—a fancy term for removal of black-heads. Didn't we just say hands off for these? Yes, but a trained facialist may be better able to remove them than you. Many states require that a skin-care specialist be trained to handle skin. In addition, a good facialist wants a return visit (or a referral or two) from you and thus is more likely to go easy on comedones, minimizing injury to skin. However, redness and blotchiness can result from extraction. Keep this in mind when scheduling a facial. The two rules good facialists live by when it comes to comedone removal: no forcing, and pressing gingerly with tissue- or cotton-reinforced fingers to buffer pressure. You may almost feel they're not trying hard enough! Best of all, of course, is extraction by a dermatologist.
- Cleansing according to skin type.
- Treatments according to skin type/skin trouble. These may include exfoliation with some scrubbing cleanser or buffing/polishing machine, a mask, an herbal pack, "nourishing" applications of collagen or elastin, electric treatments for wrinkles, pore vacuuming, etc. Here you'll find the widest variation among salons. You know how scrubs and masks work from the discussion in the at-home section of this chapter. These don't work any differently or better in a salon setting. As for electronic treatments, these painless bursts of current can cause slight surface swelling, which temporarily smooths out wrinkles. Pore vacuuming may feel effective, but nothing can get down to the bottom of a pore and clean it.
- Moisturizing according to skin type.
- Massage, often performed along with moisturizing to stimulate skin and relax you. (The only skin that should not get massaged is acne-prone skin. Stop a "pro" in mid motion if he or she attempts this, no matter what the rationale. It will not do your skin any good.) Massage may be performed during the cleansing stage, supposedly for deeper penetration of cleansers. Since you know stuff can't go any deeper than the stratum corneum, this isn't going to fool you, is it?
- Recommendation of skin-care products and makeup. One of the ironies of facials—after going to all that trouble of cleansing skin, many salons can't wait to cover it all up with makeup! To get around this, instruct your facialist to make up only your eyes, or at least to skip the foundation. Also, be forewarned: This is the big-sell step. You will be told that these products are the only ones that will "work" for your skin. If you like the smell, feel, look, and price of them, fine, buy the skin-care products. It may be a good idea to hold off until you've had other facials at other salons to compare results. However,

this can be expensive and confusing—not every salon is going to treat your skin exactly the same way.

You can expect some very real benefits from a salon facial. These include:

• A feeling of being pampered and relaxed. There's nothing wrong with this, especially since stress can show on your face. Tiny muscles tighten and accentuate existing facial wrinkles. If a salon treatment eases such signs of stress for a short time (two or three hours), there's no harm in that, is there?

• A cosmetic education. Most skin-care specialists are practiced in corrective makeup techniques or have a makeup artist on staff. They can show you how to apply makeup to camouflage a spider vein, uneven pigmentation, a scar, acne blemishes, or untreatable skin conditions.

• A cosmetic adjustment. After plastic or dermatologic surgery, you may need to make changes in the way you cleanse your skin or apply makeup.

• A new awareness of skin may also occur after a facial. You may see and experience the importance of daily care as well as preventive measures, such as wearing a sunscreen.

Skin Treatment Schedule—Professional Facials

Normal	Dry	Oily/Acne-Prone	Sensitive
As desired; skip electric treatments if pregnant.	As desired.	Blackhead extraction can redden skin; do not schedule the day before a special occasion.	Avoid steam, vacuuming, vigorous massage, electric or heat treatments.

MOISTURIZING 11

QUESTION:
  Which moisturizer should I use to help my wrinkles and lines
  go away and prevent new ones from forming?
ANSWER:
  The truth is that no moisturizer really significantly helps
  wrinkles. Moisturizers can temporarily improve the texture of
  the surface layer of skin, and that can help ease tiny surface
  crinkles. Real wrinkles come from a much deeper problem—
  deeper than any moisturizer can reach.

Five hundred million dollars is the estimated amount spent annually on moisturizers.

Most women perceive themselves as having dry facial skin. And it is no wonder, for page after page of advertisements and beauty articles imply that in endlessly repeated admonitions. Your facial skin is drying out, dryness causes wrinkles, moisturizers can clear and even prevent wrinkles, you are not beautiful unless you are *moist*, and every cosmetic and skin-care product must be moisturizing. Most of that is wrong!

The problem in this whole area of moisturizing is not that moisturizing the skin surface is a bad idea, but that the public's concept of the need for moisturizers and what moisturizers can do are so terribly incorrect. When you finish this chapter (and reread chapter 5, too) you will have a much better idea of the realities, and be a much-better-informed consumer of moisturizing products.

What moisturizers do:

Moisturizers add water to the stratum corneum and help keep it there. Remember, the stratum corneum is the tissue-paper-thin top-most layer of skin—the part of the skin that you see. Adding water to the stratum corneum makes it more flexible, less scaly, smoother-feeling, and translucent. All that adds up to "pretty."

Moisturizers do improve the look and surface texture of facial skin that suffers from surface dryness.

Moisturizers do help smooth the appearance of "tiny lines" (called crinkles in this book). This effect is most important where the skin is thinnest, the area around the eyes.

What moisturizers do not do:

Moisturizers do not penetrate deeply into the skin. They do not penetrate into the living epidermis and dermis. Indeed, they do not even penetrate very deeply into the stratum corneum. The deeper layers do not need or benefit from moisturizers—they are inside the body and *always* saturated with body fluids, *never* dry. This important fact should always be remembered when reading cosmetic and skin-care advertisements.

Moisturizers do not help real wrinkles. They only improve surface texture. Wrinkles and expression lines are a result of weakening of the deepest layer of skin, the dermis. Moisturizers put on the surface of the skin simply have no effect on these deeper layers.

Moisturizers do not prevent wrinkles. No matter what your mother or anyone else tells you, no matter what you read in cosmetic advertisements or anywhere else, *moisturizers cannot prevent wrinkles.* Protection against sun exposure is the only way to help prevent wrinkles. (There is much more on this subject in chapter 8.)

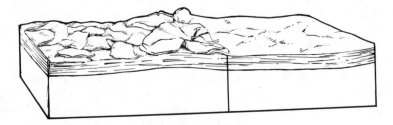

Left: Dry skin. **Right:** Moisturized skin. Note that surface cell plates are smoother on the moisturized skin, but no structural changes have occurred.

WHO SHOULD USE MOISTURIZERS

Except in the situations where they should *not* be used (see below), moisturizers are recommended anytime that skin surface dryness is a problem. The factors bearing on surface dryness are discussed in much more detail in chapter 5 (please read it!); here they are in brief:

Individual variation. Some people just have stratum corneum that cannot hold water so well—that just dries out more easily.

Low humidity. When relative humidity falls below 60 percent, stratum corneum tends to lose water to the air.

Very delicate skin is often just more comfortable when moisturizers are consistently used.

WHO SHOULD NOT USE MOISTURIZERS

Individuals who have a tendency to whiteheads, blackheads, and acne breakouts. Most moisturizers make these problems worse; some can actually cause them. Even the "oil-free" or "noncomedogenic" moisturizers are questionable. There is more about the meaning of "noncomedogenic" in chapter 14.

Individuals who have oily skin and large pores. Moisturizing this type of skin may make it feel better but causes pores to appear larger. If cleansing is not thorough, moisturizers can make the stratum corneum thicker and dull-looking.

Acne-prone skins, which are by definition oily skins, have plenty of oil in them without the addition of moisturizers. But slight surface dryness may appear even on these oily skins. It may be better to tolerate slight surface dryness then to live with a face constantly or intermittently breaking out with pimples. There is more on this subject in chapter 6.

Women with oily, acne-prone skin may of course moisturize eyelids and other non-acne-prone facial areas.

WHAT MOISTURIZER(S) TO USE

The fact is, it doesn't really matter what you use as long as you like it. All moisturizers essentially do the same thing—keep water in the stratum corneum. Some newer products—"super moisturizers"—contain special water-holding ingredients that do make them perform better.

There are about as many formulas for moisturizers as there are moisturizers, but the fundamental ingredients are:

Water, which does the moisturizing. The stratum corneum soaks up water and becomes softer, prettier, and more flexible.

Some "oil"—mineral oil, petrolatum, animal or vegetable oils, waxes, synthetic oily substances—which lies on the surface of the skin to help prevent the loss of water. The oil component does *not* soak into the stratum corneum. Your skin does not, then, absorb a moisturizer.

Emulsifying agents, which cause the water to mix with whatever oil is in the formula, so you don't have to shake a moisturizer.

Preservatives and antioxidants usually show up near the end of the ingredients list. These give the product its shelf life, but may cause skin reactions.

Special ingredients, which impart (or are advertised to impart) unique qualities to the moisturizer: collagen, aloe vera, elastin, allantoin, vitamins (A and E, mostly), lecithin, lactic acid, etc. Some are useful, others are useless. These and others are discussed in this chapter, under the heading "Super Moisturizers."

Chapter 5 has more information on moisturizers.

HOW MOISTURIZERS WORK

It may surprise you to know that skin is equipped to moisturize itself. Natural oils, or sebum, mix with perspiration on the surface of the skin to plump out dry surface cells and to form a protective layer of oil, making skin more watertight. Oily skins have more natural oils, dry (or older) skins less. Moisturizers duplicate and supplement this natural process.

Moisturizers are basically oil-in-water mixtures (or emulsions), varying in the proportions of water to oil. Cream and ointment formulas contain a high proportion of oil to water, while lotions contain more water to oil. Check the label for the order of ingredients for the relative proportions. The form the product comes in also gives you a clue: Ones with a higher oil content are thicker, usually cannot be poured, and must be scooped up with fingers. Ones with higher water content can be poured.

One on-the-spot test for oil/water concentration: Rub a bit of the product on the back of your hand. If the product contains more water than oil, you'll notice an immediate cooling sensation as some of the water evaporates. This doesn't happen with one that contains more oil than water. In fact, your hand may feel slightly warm because the oil has coated the skin. The skin will also feel more slick and have a reflective sheen to it, due to the oil.

One of the newer moisturizer formulations is labeled "oil free." Technically these products are oil free, but scan the list of ingredients and you'll find humectants, like glycerine, which help hold water in/

on the stratum corneum, and/or some synthetic oil compounds (iso-tearyl neopanteonoate, for example) that are not strictly "oils" but are oily and may be comedogenic. You can be reasonably safe in assuming that these products contain a higher water-to-oil ratio. Does that mean you can use it on acne-prone skin? That's pushing it. Better to leave acne-prone skin alone.

To review: Whatever its formulation, a moisturizer does add water to the skin. The water in water-containing products is at least partly absorbed into the stratum corneum. Other ingredients prevent the evaporative loss of water from the skin by forming a film on the surface of the skin. The heavier (the more oil, really) the moisturizer, the greater its occlusive, or water-trapping, power. In addition, some moisturizers contain water-attracting or "humectant" ingredients that bind water from the atmosphere or draw it from body tissues and hold it next to the stratum corneum. One smart-shopper tip: Don't be persuaded by claims of absorption and/or penetration. Think about it—dryness occurs on the surface layers of the stratum corneum. That's where dryness should be dealt with. You want a "superficial" moisturizer—one that stays on the surface of the stratum corneum.

DO YOU NEED SEPARATE FACE AND BODY MOISTURIZERS?

It seems that there's a lotion or some other product for just about every inch of skin—eyelids, feet, hands, breasts, body, and face. It's probably better to go by how the product feels rather than the body part named on the label. Most dermatologists tend to recommend the lighter products for facial use, except in certain conditions—ex-tremely dry skin and/or exposure to extremely drying environmental conditions.

Facial skin *is* different from body skin and may have special needs. Consider your own skin's sensitivity and needs. A very heavy body lotion may not be compatible with your facial skin. In general, facial skin has a higher oil gland concentration than arms or legs, so it may not need as heavy a product. Facial skin also tends to be a bit more reactive than body skin, so a heavily fragranced body lotion (or one high in lanolin) may irritate. Keep in mind, however, that if you are allergic to a specific ingredient, you can have a reaction on both your face and body.

If your aim is to use as few products as possible, it's best to use a moisturizer intended for the face on your body rather than vice versa. Or, for a practical, inexpensive option, try to find a light, all-purpose moisturizer, such as the following:

ALL-PURPOSE MOISTURIZERS
Nutraderm
Lubriderm
Neutrogena Moisture
Keri Lotion for Dry Skin Care
Vaseline Intensive Care
Vaseline Dermatology Formula Lotion
Nivea Moisturizing Lotion
Noxell RainTree Lotion
Sea Breeze Moisture Lotion
Youth Garde Moisturizer (plus PABA)
Moisturel
Almay Hypoallergenic Moisturizing Lotion

SHOULD YOU SWITCH MOISTURIZERS SEASONALLY?

That really depends on where you live. Obviously, skin exposed year-round to a temperate climate, with no real temperature or humidity extremes, needs no seasonal switches. If you live where winters are cold and low in humidity and the summers hot and high in humidity, the same moisturizer may not be able to meet the changing needs of your skin. Some skin-saving strategies:

1. Keep the same moisturizer and apply it to dry areas more often—after shower or bath, before bed or dressing.
2. In the fall (to prevent winter dryness), change to a more protective product (more cream than lotion). In the spring (in anticipation of summer's heat/humidity), start using a lighter product (more lotion than cream).

Two more factors to take into account: your habits and your environmental exposure. Dry skin is most often caused by a combination of really dry air and detergents or soaps that remove some of the oily protection from skin.

1. Adjust your bathing habits—take shorter baths. (Soaking in a bath for long periods of time—over fifteen minutes—can dehydrate skin further.) Or switch to taking showers—skin doesn't soak this way. You can also alternate baths with showers.
2. Use tepid water, not hot, whether you bathe or shower. Hot

water heats the skin, causing perspiration and evaporation—in other words, the loss of water to the atmosphere.

3. Switch to a soap or cleanser labeled "mild" or "for dry skin" or one containing more oil. Moisturize immediately (within two to three minutes) after bathing or showering. Bathing soaks water into skin, softening stratum corneum stiffness and roughness, and the moisturizing temporarily locks in these benefits.

4. Use a humidifier to increase the moisture content of the air. Station it in the bedroom (where you spend the most hours consecutively). A humidifier at the office isn't a bad idea either.

Such measures are not for harsh-winter areas only. If you live in a region where the humidity is high in summer, but spend most of your time indoors, your skin can dry out due to air-conditioning. You may need to adopt some of these "wintry" tactics in the heat of summer.

IS YOUR MOISTURIZER WORKING?

Product effectiveness is really a subjective call—what you feel works for you. But there are a few objective parameters:

• Try it for long enough. Give a moisturizer a trial period of about three to four weeks. During that time, cell turnover occurs—the new cells that have formed in the epidermis rise to the surface (stratum corneum), replacing old cells that have gotten rough, dry, and flaky. Of course, at the first sign of redness, itching, stinging, or swelling, product use should be discontinued, for you may have a sensitivity brewing.

• Be regular and consistent. Apply moisturizer the same number of times each day, around the same time of day. It's hard to make an informed judgment when use has been haphazard.

• Put makeup over it. Watch to see how foundation, concealer, and blusher go on . . . and stay on. A too-oily moisturizer can be at the root of streaking, fading, disappearing, or color-changing makeup.

• Skip a day. The final test of a moisturizer is to stop using it for a day. If skin still feels soft and smooth after a day off, the moisturizer is working well with your skin and personal variables such as cleansing habits and environmental exposure.

HOW TO CHOOSE A MOISTURIZER

1. Don't be swayed by the price tag. Price is not a reliable guide to the quality of a moisturizer. Outrageously expensive ones are not necessarily any better than inexpensive ones. In fact, some of the low-cost body lotions are fine facial moisturizers. What counts is how well you like the product.

2. Read the ingredients label. As you know, ingredients are listed on the label in order of descending concentration. The ingredients near the start of the list represent the largest percentage of the product. If you know your skin is sensitive to a certain ingredient, try to look for products that either do not contain the offending chemical or list it near the bottom of the list of ingredients on the package.

In general, avoid these ingredients at the top of the ingredients list if you are acne-prone:

Beeswax and other waxes
Isopropyl palmitate
Isopropyl myristate
Oleic acid
Stearic acid
Mineral oil
Lanolin, acetylated lanolin alcohol
Hydrous wool fat
Petrolatum
Spermaceti, also listed as "synthetic"
Butyl stearate
Ammonium lactate
Linseed, sesame, olive oil
Sorbitol

Avoid the following if you have sensitive skin:

Preservatives (parabens)
Lanolin, acetylated lanolin alcohol
Hydrous wool fat
Fragrances and scents
Propylene glycol

MOISTURIZERS FOR OILY/ACNE-PRONE SKIN
Drugstore Products
Wibi Lotion
Cetaphil Cream (not Lotion)
Almay Moisture Balance Lotion
Allercreme Special Formula Lotion
C&M Pharmacal Aquaderm
C&M Pharmacal Colladerm
Derma Laboratories Dermalab Cream
Sea Breeze Moisture Lotion
Complex 15 Lotion
Dermik Sherpard's Lotion
Revlon Moon Drops Moisture Film

Department Store Products
Biotherm Hydro Normaliseur
Lancôme Clarifiance
Estée Lauder Non Oily Skin Supplement

MOISTURIZERS FOR NORMAL TO DRY SKIN
Drugstore Products
Nivea Moisturizing Lotion
Vaseline Dermatology Formula
Doak Pharmaceutical Formula 405 Moisturizing Lotion
Pen-Kera (B.F. Ascher & Co.)
Revlon European Collagen Complex
Oil of Olay Beauty Lotion
Flori Roberts Melanin Moisturizer
Lohnderm Westwood Moisturel
Noxell Clarion Ultra Pure Moisturizer
Pond's Extra Rich Moisturizer Dry Skin Cream

Department Store Products
Shiseido B.H. 24 Day/Night Essence
Chanel Emulsion No. 1 Skin Equilibrium Supplement
Prescriptives Flight Cream
Biotherm Sheer Daytime Moisturizer
Lancôme Bienfait du Matin
Clinique Dramatically Different Moisturizing Lotion
Clinique Skin Texture Lotion
Clinque Very Emollient Cream
Ultima II CHR Moisture Lotion Concentrate
Lancôme Hydrix Hydrating Cream
Estée Lauder Age Controlling Creme
Christian Dior Liquid Moisture Base

SPECIALIZED MOISTURIZERS

Lip Creams

Also known as lip repair or lip fixers, these creams are variously touted for their abilities to smooth out fine lines and reduce lipstick "feathering" and "bleeding." The vertical lines above the upper lip cut through the lip margin, creating funnels for lip color to escape off the lips. They are the result of time, sun exposure, habits (smoking), and expression (puckering and pursing of lips).

Basically, these products cause a temporary swelling of the skin above the lip, so lines seem to fill in. They also contain fixatives to keep lip color in place. It's the fixative, preventing the creep of color and lipstick, that really offers a solution to this problem.

AT-HOME ALTERNATIVES TO LIP-FIX PRODUCTS

- Use a moisturizer in the area above the lips. It's one of the most overlooked areas for moisturizing. Now, as you well know, a moisturizer will not "cure" wrinkles, but it will affect skin dryness, which makes lines more obvious.
- Use a sunscreen in this area. You won't recoup any breakdown of collagen that caused the lines, but you'll stop them from getting any worse.
- Apply loose powder to lips and just outside the lip border—it forms a stable base for makeup and keeps lip liner from blurring.
- Line lips with a lip pencil. A lip pencil is just lipstick with a high paraffin (wax) content. The wax discourages bleeding. After you've finished lining lips, gently whisk away any excess powder from around the mouth with a small makeup brush.
- Fill in lips with matching lip color, but only to the edge of the pencil line, not on top of it. Lip colors labeled "long-lasting" may be a good choice. To get hours-longer staying power, they are formulated with less emollient. The less greasy the product, the less likely it is to migrate.

Eye Creams

These creams have the same basic formula as moisturizers, but have more oil, usually in the form of wax, to help minimize smaller crinkles. One side effect you don't hear about—the number of sensitivity reactions. Eyelid skin is the thinnest on the body, and reaction can show up here first. Possible troublemakers: the scents, the preservatives, and even some of the ingredients. The problems they claim to solve—reducing puffiness and smoothing out wrinkles—can successfully be addressed with other products. Gel-filled eye compresses, available in most drugstores, can de-puff swollen eyes via cooling. And your regular facial moisturizer will probably substitute nicely for an eye cream. One application tip: Dot moisturizer an inch away from eyes, so you don't accidentally put cream in them and cause temporarily cloudy vision or stinging. Body heat will cause just the right amount of the product to migrate toward the eye.

Night Creams

Night creams contain more oil than most daytime moisturizers. Applying a heavy moisturizer at night seems to be a long-standing beauty practice. Your mother may have done it to try to prevent wrinkles. However, it is a fact that soaking facial skin overnight in a heavy greasy moisturizer will not cure wrinkles.

Still, the myth is perpetuated. Many cosmetic lines feature an overnight moisturizing product as the star of the show. That product is almost always the most expensive item in the line, and almost always is the greasiest. (The advertising euphemism is "rich".)

Guidelines for using an overnight moisturizer. Use one if you wish. Do not use one if you tend to have acne breakouts. Don't feel you have to use a moisturizer specifically labeled for such a purpose—your day moisturizer may work just fine. An overnight moisturizer doesn't have to be greasy; a light one is certainly adequate (especially if you've got a humidifier going) and may be more cosmetically acceptable. It may save you from having to wash grease stains off your pillowcase! Finally, don't feel compelled to spend big money for an expensive overnight product. Inexpensive ones may be just as good for your skin. Want something heavy, "rich," and not at all pricey? Try cold cream.

"Super" Moisturizers

A step beyond regular moisturizers are the super moisturizers. Along with the standard water-and-oil formulations most of these have an added ingredient that boosts moisturizing performance by holding water in and on the skin's surface. These additions do help . . . but probably not as much as the hype. Just remember that, super or not, no matter what they contain, moisturizers moisturize the thin lifeless top layer of skin—not the deeper layers. For a review of these ingredients, refer to chapter 7. Here are the major additives:

Collagen, procollagen, hydrolized collagen. This protein, which occurs naturally in the body's connective tissue, forms a gel with water, and this film holds water against the stratum corneum. Collagen is especially good at binding water to the outer layer of skin in lower humidity. Some products that contain collagen:

Department Store Products
Ultima II ProCollagen Skin Repair
Revlon European Collagen Complex
Estée Lauder Non-Oily Skin Supplement
Estee Lauder Swiss Performing Extract
Clinique Skin Texture Lotion
Ultima II ProCollagen Anti-Aging Complex for Face

Drugstore Products
Pond's Cream and Collagen
St. Ives Swiss Formula with Collagen & Elastin

Elastin and other proteins, amino acids. Elastin is another body protein, found interwoven between collagen fibers in the skin. It is thought to play a role in making the skin supple and flexible. It, as well as other proteins, also forms gels in the presence of water. Amino acids are the building blocks of proteins and so share some of the same characteristics. Some products that contain these:

Department Store Products
Lancôme Progres Plus Creme Anti-Rides
Chanel Skin Regeneration Treatment
Discipline Pro Cell-T
Clinique Sub-Skin Cream
Germaine Monteil Supplegen Firming Action Moisture Cream

Drugstore Products
St. Ives Swiss Formula with Collagen & Elastin

Mucopolysaccharides (another group of water binders)

Department Store Products
Germaine Monteil Supplegen Instant Action Firmer

Chondroitin sulfate

Department Store Products
Avon Night Support

Hyaluronic acid

Department Store Products
Sebastian Cellular Day Care
Sebastian Cellular Night Care
Estée Lauder Night Repair Cellular Recovery Complex
Avon Night Support
Shiseido Facial Concentrates

Glycosphingolipid

Department Store Products
Glycel (Altin)

Drugstore Products
Revlon Eterna 27 All-Day Moisture Cream

Aloe (a plant extract that may have some water-binding capacity)

Department Store Products
Estée Lauder Age Controlling Cream

Drugstore Products
Fran Wilson Collagen Elastin with Aloe Vera
Avon Care Deeply
Vaseline Intensive Care Lotion with Aloe
Bonne Bell Moisture Lotion

Lactic acid, glycolic acid (alpha-hydroxy acids), and urea. These additives may boost the moisture-holding capacity of a product, but they also tend to remove dead surface skin cells, giving skin a smoother look and feel. These additives may cause a stinging sensation, especially on the face.

LACTIC ACID
Drugstore Products
Lacticare Lotion
Lac-Hydrin (prescription only)
Fran Wilson Collagen Elastin with Aloe Vera
Purpose Dry Skin Cream

Department Store Products
Prescriptives Flight Cream

GLYCOLIC ACID
Drugstore Products
Aquaglycolic Lotion

UREA
Drugstore Products
Coty Overnight Success Cellular Replacement Cream
Nutraplus Cream and Lotion
Aquacare and Aquacare H.P. Cream and Lotion

Phospholipids. These are also components of skin surface cells and are thought to play a major role in holding water in the skin surface. We know that dryness of the skin surface is at least partly due to a loss of phospholipids. Adding these compounds to moisturizers does seem to help. Studies show that the use of a phospholipid moisturizer seems to keep the skin surface from drying out again so quickly.

Lecithin. This is a phospholipid derived from soy beans. Each molecule of this substance is capable of holding fifteen molecules of water, making it an effective binder on the skin surface. Products that contain one or the other of these:

Drugstore Products
Complex Moisturizing 15 Face Cream
Mary Kay Night Cream for Dry Skin

Ascorbic Acid (Vitamin C). Vitamin C is essential for the production of collagen in the deeper layers of the skin. The addition of ascorbic acid to moisturizing products may help in skin collagen production and thus help in repairing the deeper skin deterioration that causes wrinkles. At the time of this writing, we do not know if it really works, but it does sound like a good idea. We know of only one product that is currently on the market: Avon Collagen Booster.

FACIAL SKIN COSMETICS

Foundations, Blushers, and Powders

12

QUESTION:
> If I use expensive cosmetic products, am I taking better care of
> my skin than if I use inexpensive ones?

ANSWER:
> No. Price is not guide to the quality of a skin-care or cosmetic
> product. Price is governed by packaging and advertising costs
> and the market segment at which the product is aimed. The
> vast majority of cosmetic and skin-care products maintain high
> standards of quality and purity, no matter what the price
> range.

WHAT PRICE BEAUTY?

Does beauty have a price? It certainly seems to when it comes to
makeup . . . and the price always seems so high! The good news is
that cost has little, if anything, to do with the clinical effectiveness—
the results—of any cosmetic. If you want to spend more for a
product—because you like the shade, the packaging, the brand name,
the cachet/fantasy of owning a "designer" cosmetic—go ahead. But
please don't feel pressured into buying it. There are plenty of lower-
priced products that are just as effective.

While shopping for low- or no-frills cosmetics means you give up
the "trained" sales help found in the department stores, manufacturers
of products sold in drugstores and outlets are trying to steer you right.
Clarion, a skin-care and cosmetic line from Noxell, furnishes a
"computer" that suggests products based on the customer's skin color
and skin type. Another drugstore standard, Max Factor, has developed
packaging that "codes" or groups appropriate products by skin type.

95

FOUNDATION MAKEUP

These products have the sole purpose of making skin look prettier—by covering small imperfections, smoothing out skin-color tones, giving skin a "finish." Skillfully used, they do these things beautifully. You wind up with the appearance of skin with a finer texture, a subtle luster, perhaps a hint of heightened color.

Basically, a foundation contains water, oil, pigment, and various waxes. They are available in an endless variety of colors and formulas—hypoallergenic, scented, unscented, fragrance-free, oil-free, water-based, moisturizing, oil-controlling, and goodness knows what else. You can buy liquid, cream, cake, crayon, and mousse types. The form you choose is a matter of personal perference—it's the one you feel you can control, that gives you the results you want.

There is also an enormous price range. Make no mistake about it, though, the inexpensive ones are just as good for you as the expensive ones. The major cosmetics manufacturers all produce products of high quality and purity. There are few exceptions to this. So do not feel you have to spend a lot for a good foundation makeup.

Having said that, it is also necessary to point out that *any* of these products may cause problems (see chapter 16, "Adverse Reactions to Cosmetics"), but such problems are really relatively rare. Essentially, all cosmetics marketed by major manufacturers have a low potential for allergy and irritancy, whether or not they are labeled "hypoallergenic."

FOUNDATION GUIDELINES

The million-dollar question: Which foundation to use? The advice here is simple: Choose the one that appeals to you. From a skin-health perspective, here are a few guidelines, according to skin type:

Opt for Lighter Coverage

No matter what your skin type, remember—lighter, less greasy products give a more natural look to skin. Foundations should be used to blend and tone rather than to plaster over and cover the skin completely. Lighter foundations are also less prone to cause problems with whiteheads, blackheads, and breakouts.

Finally, lighter, less greasy products are much easier to remove completely in facial cleansing.

How to find a "light" foundation? Read the label. All foundations are about half water, so water is usually the first ingredient listed, look beyond this to the rest of the list. A foundation with more oils in its listing is going to be heavier. One with more filler or thickener (such as talc, clay, zinc oxide, or aluminum silicate) is going to be lighter. Read the buzz words—"translucent," "sheer," "matte," "natural," "light" are all tip-offs to a lighter formula.

HOW GREASY IS YOUR FOUNDATION? A TEST

To find a light, as-greaseless-as-possible foundation, use this easy test to try before you buy. Take a sheet of bond paper (at least 25 percent cotton rag) to the makeup counter. Using the store testers, dab a bit of several different foundations on the paper. Label each dab carefully. Place the paper in a dry protected place. Check it a day later for signs of an oil ring. Any oil in the product will migrate out from the dab, absorbed by the paper. The larger the ring, the greater the amount of oil in the product. Buy the one with the smallest ring.

Guidelines for Dry Skin

Older skin or dry skin may need a creamier foundation formula for the best coverage. Ones with a higher water content may not have enough "slip," or lubrication, to go on evenly to suit these skin types. That doesn't mean heading for the heaviest, oiliest base in the store. Instead, find the lightest one that gives you coverage. Lighter products are crucial for dry or older skins—too heavy a product can accentuate crinkles, lines, and wrinkles. Don't use foundation to spackle in facial lines—it just can't be done. Look for emollients or oils (usually mineral oil) in the ingredients listing; for the buzzwords "moist" and "dewy"; and/or for claims of coverage. (The more oil in a formula, the more coverage it provides . . . and the more heavily it goes on skin. Other covering agents are titanium dioxide, talc, and kaolin. If you want more coverage, look for these near the top of the ingredients list.) What if "moist" or "dewy" is just too shiny for you and "matte" is too dry? A good compromise is the semimatte formula, which gives a nice finish with just a bit of shine, or "radiance" as it's often referred to on labels.

Another option: Apply your usual moisturizer before applying a lighter foundation. The moisturizer underlayer may provide just the amount of emollient slip needed for a good result. There are also tinted moisturizers available that give skin a sheer color, so you can skip foundation altogether.

FOUNDATIONS FOR DRY SKIN
Drugstore Products
Helena Rubinstein Liquid Silk Foundation
Revlon Natural Wonder "Fresh-All-Day" Moisturizing Makeup
Almay Protectives Skin Care for Age Control Lasting Finish Liquid Makeup
Max Factor Ultralucent Moisturizing Pure Moisture Fluid Make-Up
Maybelline Mousse Make-up
Allercreme Satin Finish Makeup
Almay Fresh Glow Moisture Makeup

Department Store Products
Ultima II Actives Protective Face Color Mousse
Clarins Revitalizing Tinted Moisturizer
Ultima II ProCollagen Anti-Aging Firming Foundation

Guidelines for Normal Skin

This is the skin that most often has more defined drier areas (cheeks) combined with oilier ones (nose, chin, forehead), so it's best to choose a foundation that works on both. Try foundations that are mostly water (with oil appearing toward the middle of the ingredients list), or look for one that contains oil blotters (label buzz words include "minimizing" and "oil-controlling"). A sheer formulation may be fine for drier areas, but you may notice that it won't quite hide broken capillaries, large pores, or uneven skin tone in oilier areas. In that case, look for one that gives light to medium coverage.

FOUNDATIONS FOR NORMAL SKIN
Drugstore Products
L'Erin Moisture Fresh Makeup
Max Factor Creme Puff Makeup
Almay Maximum Protection Cream-Powder Makeup

Department Store Products
Lancôme Bienfait du Matin Multi-Protective Day Cream
Clinique Face Zone Sun Block
Biotherm Teint Tonic Protective Moisturizer
Clinique Balanced Makeup Base
Chanel Teint Naturel Liquid Makeup
Shiseido Moisture Mist Liquid Foundation
Lancôme Maquimat Teint Naturel

Clarin's Revitalizing Tinted Moisturizer
Ultima II ProCollagen Anti-Aging Firming Foundation
Estée Lauder Polished Performance Liquid Makeup
Lancôme Dual Finish Cream/Powder Makeup
Estée Lauder Fresh Air Makeup Base

FOUNDATIONS WITH SUNSCREEN

Fair-skinned, light-eyed individuals do need daily sun protection, so foundations containing sunscreens would seem to be a great idea. However, most foundations labeled "contains sunscreen" are not labeled with a SPF number, although a few exceptions do exist.

Instead of taking your chances with unlabeled SPF-containing foundations, why not apply sunscreen under your foundation as part of your makeup routine. Twenty years from now, you'll thank us!

Guidelines for Oily and/or Acne-Prone Skin

Individuals with active acne usually want heavy coverage to hide the problem. Much better advice is to treat the problem (see specific pointers in chapter 14). Choose a medium-coverage foundation and apply it over blemishes that have been dabbed first with a medicated coverup for the most natural-looking effect. Trying to hide blemishes with makeup can make pimples worse.

It's worth repeating: The wrong foundation may cause breakout problems on clear faces and aggravate these problems on breakout-prone faces. Very frequently, dermatologists consult with women who are using the wrong foundation and are having skin trouble as a result.

It is difficult for an acne-prone person to read labels and to decide on a foundation that won't cause problems; because, unfortunately, makeup labeling is misleading or inconclusive. And when it comes to acne-prone skin, the wrong product has long-lasting skin consequences . . . blemishes. Terms such as "oil-free," "water-based," "oil control," "hypoallergenic," and "dermatologist-tested" do not necessarily mean that a foundation is safe for acne-prone skin. Even the new phrase "noncomedogenic," advertised to mean it cannot cause breakouts, may not be safe for the acne-prone face. While such a product may contain no animal or vegetable fats (known acne aggravators), they contain synthetic oil derivatives to make them moist and easier to apply. These can cause problems in some people.

Surprisingly, foundations that contain alcohol may be too drying for skin if used in conjunction with a very drying acne medication.

FOUNDATIONS FOR OILY/ACNE-PRONE SKIN
Drugstore Products
Almay Fresh Look Oil Free Makeup
Almay Smart Cover Makeup
Helena Rubinstein Bio-Clear
Revlon Natural Wonder Oil Free Base
Allercreme Matte Finish
Maybelline Shine Free Oil Control Dual Powder Base
Cover Girl Oily Control Make-Up

Department Store Products
Lancôme Macquicontrôle Oil-Free Liquid Make-Up
Clinique Workout Makeup
Janet Sartin Day Wear Astringent
Germaine Monteil Visage Clarité
Ultima II Formula 2 Makeup
Elizabeth Arden Extra Control for Oily Skin
Clinique Pore Minimizer Makeup
Prescriptives Oil Free Exact Color Makeup
Estée Lauder Oil Control Formula
Erno Lazlo Normalizing "Shake It" Foundation

Guidelines for Sensitive Skin

This skin type needs the lightest possible coverage ("sheer," "translucent") or, if you can get away with it, no foundation at all (see the section on powders on page 104). Products labeled "unscented and fragrance-free" are a good bet. Possible irritants include perfumes, oils, starchy fillers, preservatives, and propylene glycol surfactants (sodium laurel sulfate, for example). Even formulas labeled "hypoallergenic" are no guarantee of nonirritancy. One more skin troubler to be on the lookout for is sunscreen. The most common chemical, PABA, is a known skin irritant and sensitizer. Plus, as has already been mentioned, a foundation containing sunscreen does not usually bear an SPF number, so you don't know how much (or how little) protection you're actually getting. A PABA-free sunscreen (SPF 15 or higher) applied before foundation is a better bet.

FOUNDATIONS FOR SENSITIVE SKIN
Drugstore Products
Almay Moisturizing Foundation
Allercreme Matte Finish, Velvet Finish and Satin Finish Makeup
Noxell Clarion Foundation

Department Store Products
Clinique Balanced Makeup Base
Estée Lauder Soft Finish Compact Makeup

Helpful hint: To get the thinnest, most even coverage, it's important to use the right tools. For the standard, drier, oil-free formulas, which have neither as much slip, nor as much "play time" (the time a product remains moist and spreadable, allowing the user time to "play" or arrange it to her satisfaction before it dries), a moistened cosmetic sponge is key to giving you the result you want.

GOOF PROOFING YOUR FOUNDATION SHOPPING

• *Test products in the store with conditions as close as possible to how you would do it at home.* Before you leave the house to foundation shop, wash your face and apply moisturizer, or whatever else you would do before applying foundation. This way, when you try a product on in the store, you can better gauge how it looks on your face.

• *Choose the right color.* Test foundation shades on the jawline—it's easy to see in the mirror, and there are no features to cast a shadow and "color" your evaluation. The one that seems to disappear into surrounding skin is the one for you. The only difference between the sample and your skin should be smoothness. A distinct line means it's too dark; a chalky appearance means it's too light. Can't find a perfect match? Err a bit on the yellow side. Foundations with pink or orange tones in them can look artificial or just plain gray on skin.

• *Choose the right consistency for your skin type.* Consistency determines how smoothly and finely a product applies. For example, a mostly water foundation may dry too quickly or may not have enough slip to apply evenly to dry skin. The best place to test for a consistency match is the inside of your wrist. See how easily it applies, how thinly it can be spread over the skin.

Applying Foundation

Use the right tools to apply foundation. A dense synthetic latex or cosmetic sponge (it may also be called a "silk" sponge) or a small natural sea sponge gives the most natural results. Dampen the sponge first, then apply the product.

You probably know that you should dot foundation onto forehead, nose, chin, and cheeks, but did you know you should apply these dots to one area at a time, blending thoroughly before dotting the next area? Premature dotting allows the product to dry out, and it may not blend as well. Blend using light outward and upward strokes. If you notice any streaks or uneven areas once this process is completed, don't apply more foundation. Redampen the sponge (it should feel barely damp) and smooth over these areas.

Ever wonder just how much a dot of foundation is? When you touch your finger to your face, it should leave a mark of foundation that's about the size of an M & M.

BLUSHERS

For color in the cheeks, for toning makeup, and for highlighting and contouring the cheekbones, blushers add the finishing touch. They are available in cream, gel, powder, soft crayon/pencil, and mousse forms.

The only caution here applies to those with oily or acne-prone skin, for some blushers may cause blackheads, whiteheads, and sometimes pimples in the blush zone.

There are a few things to consider here. First, the cream blushers (which have an oily or waxy base) are more likely to cause pore problems than powder types. Even gel types (which are petrolatum-based) can kick up problems.

The red dyes in the blusher (usually D&C #11 or #17) may do the same thing. It is difficult to say just how important a problem this is, but if changing from a cream blush to a dry powder does not solve your blocked-pore woes, try a powder eye shadow as a blusher. The pinkish shades of eye powder contain a different red dye—one that is less likely to cause breakout problems.

Remember, too, that some products contain fragrances, lanolin, or preservatives that can cause a skin reaction.

The Four Biggest Blush Mistakes

Correct these and you'll get a natural, fresh look from blush.

1. *Applying blush in a straight-line streak.* This approach is much too harsh for any face. The right shape is a "pork chop"—widest at the front of the face, tapering back and up toward the outer brow. The edges of this "pork chop" should be softly blended so there is no noticeable demarcation line.

2. *Misusing—or not using—the proper blush applicator.* Applying blush with the right tool helps achieve both the right shape and the right degree of blending. A triangular wedge sponge is used for gel,

Blushers

Blush Type	Skin Type	Comments
Powder	All skin types, especially oily	Can "turn" on oily skins Easiest to work with Covers small imperfections Apply over foundation and over powder
Gel (also color wash, color rub, stain)	Dry, older skins	Gives sheer finish but dries rapidly Needs frequent reapplication Watch for blocked pores Apply over foundation and under powder
Cream	Dry, older skins	Longest-lasting form Apply over foundation and under powder
Mousse	All types except acne-prone	Watch for blocked pores Apply over foundation and under powder
Crayon/pencil	Trouble-free	Long-lasting Can drag or pull on application Apply over foundation and under powder

cream, mousse, and pencil types. For cream or gel blushes, rub the wider end over the blush, then blot on the back of your hand to blend the color and remove any excess. Stipple it onto your cheeks quickly, then blend with the narrower end. For mousse blushes, dispense a dime-sized amount into your palm and blend with the fingers until creamy. Apply with the fingers and blend with the wedge sponge. For crayon types, apply with the pencil tip and blend with sponge.

Blush brushes are used for powder blushes. Don't use the applicator that comes with powder blush—it's too thin and flat to give good results. The right brush has dense bristles at least 2½ inches long, cut in a dome shape that forms a 2-inch-wide fan when pressed against the skin. Soft bristles (sable or squirrel), not coarse ones (such as pony), are less irritating to the skin and also distribute the blush more evenly. Run the brush over the surface of the blush, and tap or blow off the excess before applying it to your face.

Money-saving tip: Buy blush brushes in an art supply store. That way, you're not paying extra for a company name. Ask for artist's or potter's brushes.

3. *Applying blush to the front of the face only.* This can close in a face. Remember, your face is three-dimensional. Blusher should be applied along the natural curve of the cheekbone, all the way to the hairline. Proper use of blush (combined with the right tool) can give it depth and definition.

4. *Choosing too dark a shade.* The most common error is assuming that the darker the blush, the longer it will last. Wrong. In fact, too dark a shade can actually make your cheekbones recede! Match blush to your skin tone:

Skin Tone	Blush Shade
Ivory to beige	Pinks
Olive	Peaches and corals
Dark, black	Rusts and spices

FACIAL POWDERS

To "set" foundation and blush, to create a matte (no-shine) finish, and to reduce oily sheen, reach for a face powder. Once considered "grandmotherly," powders are popular again because, used properly, they give skin a clean finish. In fact, they have become a foundation alternative. Powders are fine for all skin types to use. For oily skin, look for a product high in talc or chalk to mop up excess oil. Dry skin types can use ones that contain more oil or claim to be moisturizing.

The basic formula for a loose powder is a base (talcum, clay, magnesium silicate, magnesium almuminum silicate), spreading/adhering/covering agents (kaolin, silicone, zinc stearate), pigments, preservatives, and perfumes. Pressed powders contain an oil or gum to hold the ingredients together.

You can choose from neutral (no color) powders or tinted powders, also known as "full-coverage" powders. Brand new on the scene is a foundation/powder hybrid. A blend of cream foundation and powder in a compact, these products can be applied with a damp sponge for a moist foundation effect or dry for a matte powder effect. While the choice is yours, these products are heavier—a wet application can result in a pancake effect. Try the dry application—it yields a more natural finish but covers enough to eliminate the need for foundation.

Tips for Powder Perfection

• Opt for loose rather than pressed powders. A loose powder contains more air, so it's easier to apply lightly. Pick one that is labeled "translucent"—it lets your natural skin color show through. You'll use less, and less is healthier for skin.

• Apply with clean soft brush—soft so it doesn't irritate skin and clean because a buildup of skin oils on bristles can cause the powder to turn an off color. Needless to say, brushes should be stored in a makeup bag, not let loose in a purse, and should never be lent or borrowed, as infections can be spread.

• Apply powder with sweeping motions, from the center of the face out toward the hairline.

• Finish by buffing away the excess. To achieve a delicate, transparent effect, take a clean brush or cotton ball and gently smooth over the powder with small circular motions.

• For pressed powders, press the powder into place; don't rub a puff over the skin. Don't store the puff in the compact; skin oils can accumulate and turn powder an off color. Best to toss the puff and use cotton balls.

• Money-saving tip: Good old Johnson & Johnson Baby Powder is an inexpensive alternative to face powder. In spite of the fact that it is white, when properly applied and buffed with brushes, it leaves a great translucent finish on skin.

POWDERS
Drugstore Products
Coty Correctives Powder
Maybelline Shine Free Oil Control Dual Base Powder
Max Factor Ultralucent Ultra Sheer Face Powder
Cover Girl Translucent Blotting Powder
Almay Translucent Finish Face Powder
Revlon Skin Balancing Powder Creme Makeup
Almay Shine Free Blotting Powder

Department Store Products
Shiseido Moisture Mist Compact Foundation
Chanel Poudre Douce
Lancôme Boite A Poudre
Alexandra de Markoff Finishing Powder
Lancôme MacquiFinish Pressed Powder Translucent Mat

COSMETIC CAMOUFLAGE—HOW TO HIDE WHAT YOU HATE

Makeup not only plays up great skin, it can help conceal skin flaws and transient facial crises. Here's a rundown of the most common:

Undereye circles. Use a concealer (a cream or stick product that is more opaque than foundation) in a shade lighter than your skin (or foundation). Don't cover the whole undereye area—this may only accentuate the problem. Apply only to the dark circle, using a small flat brush, then apply foundation.

Large pores. Less makeup is the key to minimizing large pores. Apply a sheer matte foundation and blend it subtly, using a wedge sponge. Top with loose translucent powder. Be sure to buy a fine-milled powder. A coarse one can exaggerate pore size. Test powder by rubbing it between the thumb and index finger—a finely milled product should feel silky, with no distinct graininess.

Acne. Disguise a blemish by dabbing on a medicated coverup (such as Clearasil Tinted Cream or Stick, Owen Lab's Liquimat Lotion, Clinique Anti Acne Control Formula, or Shiseido Pureness Spot Cream). Be sure to dab the coverup right on the very top of the pimple, not the surrounding tissue. On unblemished skin, these medicated products cause dryness and flakiness—more unsightliness. Then cover with foundation. Don't use a regular concealer—the oils contained in it could make the blemish worse.

To tone down allover rednesss, try a green-toned primer under foundation. Adrien Arpel Porcelain Cover Base, Shiseido Green Moisture Mist Compact Foundation, Countess Isserlyn Tuna Cover Base, and Marcella Borghese Velluto Liquid Toner Verde are all good. Apply sparingly, and blot well with a tissue. These are a bit on the oily side, and overdoing it could raise another bump.

Acne scars. Light casts shadows in the depressions left by acne or other injuries. Use a stick concealer and gently roll the color into the skin depression. Smooth out with foundation. Or mix a bit of loose powder into your usual foundation for a matte, heavier makeup. Spot-apply to scars. Keep makeup finishes matte—luminescent finishes can highlight imperfections.

Broken blood vessels. These little squiggly red lines are actually enlarged, not broken, vessels. Most of the time, an extra dab of foundation is all that's needed to cover them up. For especially large or red vessels, use a green toned primer, as discussed above. Apply it to the area with your fingers, using short strokes. Buff with a cotton ball to blend in the edges. Apply foundation. For more on these, see chapter 19.

Undereye crinkles, lines. Avoid concealers in this area—their heavier formula tends to settle into lines and accentuate them. Instead, mix half moisturizer and half foundation in the palm of one hand. Pat on with a fingertip. Then take a fine makeup sponge and roll it back and forth to blot the excess. Dust with powder to set coverup.

Corner-of-eye crinkles, lines. To soften crow's feet, brush in a bit of pale powder. The pale color lightens the dark of the crease, visually flattening it. Apply eye makeup toward the center of eye to direct attention away from corners and also to lessen any clumping of shadow in creases.

FIXING WRINKLES

13

QUESTION:
I've read this whole book up to here, and I think I understand about my skin and about skin-care products. I'm getting wrinkles, and I need guidance. Can you help me?
ANSWER:
Maybe. This chapter takes you through the various options for dealing with wrinkles and helps you decide what might really work for you.

The search for a medicine, skin-care product, or process that really will remove wrinkles goes on—and now more feverishly than ever. Just read the skin-care advertisements and beauty columns in a couple of popular magazines, and you will surely be convinced.

Before reading this, please be sure you have read chapters 3, 5, 7, and 11.

The primary cause of real wrinkles is sun damage to the dermis—the deepest, thickest, and strongest layer of skin. The cause of crinkles or "tiny lines" is dryness of the skin surface. This surface dryness does also contribute to the appearance of real wrinkles.

Age—usually age of fifty-plus years—causes more thinning and weakening of the dermis, and more tendency to surface dryness. Thus, age, sun damage, and dry skin surface all play a role in wrinkling.

Sun damage to the dermis seems to be the most important factor, for the dermis is the thickest, strongest layer of skin. Make that layer thinner and weaker (that's what sun exposure does) and you have wrinkles. Weakened skin constantly stretched and creased by facial expression can't recover its shape and just stays creased.

Skin surface dryness causes the tissue-paper-thin stratum corneum to shrink—pulling weakened, sun-damaged skin into crinkles, or "tiny lines." This is a major factor where skin is thinnest—around and below the eyes.

Deep expression lines such as brow furrows, frown lines, and smile lines around the mouth are caused by habitual facial expressions with sun damage making them all the worse.

WRINKLE-REMOVING OPTIONS

Option I: Moisturizers

Using a moisturizer—expensive or inexpensive—smooths, softens, and relaxes the stratum corneum. Moisturizing helps erase tiny lines that come from skin surface dryness and helps improve surface texture. But moisturizing does simply nothing for real wrinkles—those that come from the sun-damaged dermis.

Choose this option if your problem is crinkles from surface dryness. Chapter 11 contains a list of good products.

Option II: Super Moisturizers

Moisturizer enhancers such as protein, collagen, procollagen, elastin, mucopolysaccharides, chondroitin sulfate, hyaluronic acid, glycosphingolipid, aloe, and phospholipids simply help a moisturizing product hold water in the skin's thin top layer better. They boost a moisturizer's performance. As with plain moisturizers, they affect only the thin top layer of skin and do essentially nothing for the dermis, where real wrinkles are.

Moisturizers with urea added also bind water to the stratum corneum better. An extra plus to urea-containing products is that they also help remove dead surface cell plates, thereby giving skin a brighter look. Urea may cause stinging on sensitive faces.

Moisturizers with alpha-hydroxy acids (the so-called fruit acids), such as glycolic, lactic, malic, citric, tartaric, and gluconic acids, deserve special mention. At the time of this writing there is increasing interest in these substances as wrinkle fighters. It is thought that the major effect of these substances is on that thin top layer of skin where other moisturizers also work, but there is a difference. Alpha-hydroxy acids exert a powerful force in removing dead surface cell plates—even to the extent of removing thin surface growths and spots and unblocking blocked pores. Initial studies have shown good effects on surface crinkles. More study is needed to find out if these effects are long-lasting and if any beneficial changes are occurring deeper in the skin, where real wrinkles are.

Products now available contain lactic or glycolic acids. They are listed in chapter 11. One problem with these ingredients is that they often cause stinging on sensitive faces.

Choose this option if your problem is surface dryness and crinkling and you are interested in spending a good deal more to get something that is more effective than a regular moisturizer. Products in this category are listed in chapter 11.

Option III: Moisturizers with Sunscreen Ingredients

You have read about this in many places in this book. Sunscreen products do help protect the skin from wrinkling. Sunscreen products with a high level of protection (SPF 15 or higher) should be used all the time, beginning early in life. They will not cure wrinkles or "reverse the signs of aging." A product labeled "sunscreen added" is not good enough—make sure you use a product with that SPF 15 or higher on the package.

Option IV: Retinoic Acid

This potent active chemical (found only in products available with a physician's prescription) is the most promising substance in the search for the fountain of youth. Retinoic acid has effects on both the upper and deeper layers of skin. In the topmost stratum corneum layer it helps in the removal of lifeless cell plates; in the epidermis it speeds cell renewal rate and pigment dispersal; and in the deepest dermis layer it promotes the growth of new blood vessels and the production of new collagen fibers.

It is a drug, not a cosmetic. It really does help skin renew itself.

It is wiser to think of retinoic acid as a means of slowing down the skin aging process than as a wrinkle remover, though some real and important rebuilding of sun-damaged skin may occur. The use of retinoic acid may even out pigment splotches and may prevent some forms of skin cancer. Long-term use (years) is required for all these effects to occur.

Sounds good? Right, but retinoic acid is tricky to use. It is a strong skin irritant and should be used only under the guidance of a skilled dermatologist. Otherwise, you may get a red, peeling, unhappy face. Consult your dermatologist about whether it is appropriate for your skin.

Choose this option especially if your eyes are blue or green, your complexion is fair, and your skin is wrinkled from too much sun exposure. It is an important breakthrough. More about it in chapter 7.

Option V: Ascorbic Acid

Ascorbic acid—that's vitamin C to you—is critical to the skin's ability to manufacture collagen. And you know that collagen fibers form the strength and framework of the deepest layer of skin. So why not put ascorbic acid in a skin cream so that it will penetrate into the dermis and improve collagen synthesis? Well, they are doing that right now. The product now available is Avon Collagen Booster.

At the time of this writing, no good clinical experiments have been done on wrinkled faces using ascorbic acid creams. By the time you read this, there may have been. You will certainly be hearing more about it.

Ascorbic acid is not very stable in solution (it may tend to break down and lose effectiveness) and does not penetrate very well to the deeper layers of skin where it needs to be to do some good. These problems may be solved, though, and ascorbic acid may become an important ingredient in the struggle against wrinkles.

Option VI: Plastic Surgery and Wrinkle-Filling Injections

Plastic surgeons and some dermatologists can work wonders with cosmetic surgical techniques. For badly wrinkled facial skin, a consultation with one of these specialists is definitely in order. Collagen and other materials can be injected into facial skin to elevate and remove individual wrinkles and lines. Dermabrasion or chemical peeling may be done to remove wrinkles and give facial skin a whole new surface. Surgical face lifting and eyelid surgery can remove excess sagging skin and tighten up the facial areas that need it.

For a badly wrinkled face, these procedures can do what no cosmetic or skin-care product can do. Do investigate this option if you have badly wrinkled skin.

PART THREE

Skin Problems

BREAKOUT PROBLEMS
Acne

For those of you whose face just never outgrew the acne years, having breakout problems past the teenage years and even into your thirties and forties is still the same old annoying thing.

But for those of you who never had teenage acne or who had some teenage acne problems and outgrew them, it is a real shock to start having breakouts in the mid twenties to late thirties.

This is not shocking to dermatologists; they are consulted frequently by women well past their teenage years who have acne problems. Statistics support the notion that adult acne is a very common problem—50 percent of the females who consult dermatologists about acne are in the twenty-five- to forty-five-year-old group. And many dermatologists feel that this problem is on the increase. It needs to be understood better by those women who have it.

Adult acne can usually be controlled with proper skin care and the intelligent use of over-the-counter medications. And, if that is not enough, dermatologists have expertise and access to prescription medications that will certainly help.

Let us define our terms in the way that dermatologists do. Do you really have acne, or just little breakouts? The word "acne" conjures up a picture of a really bad complexion problem, but it should not. Dermatologists use the term "acne" to cover a broad range of complexion problems, from the very minor to the very severe.

ACNE LESIONS

Blackheads (open comedones) are visibly enlarged pores filled with a plug of dead skin cells and skin oil. The top of a blackhead is often dark, but in blonds and redheads it may be light-colored.

Whiteheads (closed comedones, milia) are, like blackheads, a compacted mass of dead skin cells and skin oil in a pore. But the top is closed by a thin layer of skin. They are just little white bumps under the surface, best seen by slightly stretching the skin.

Pustules, pimples. These are small inflamed (red) bumps with pus in the top.

Papules, pimples. Another small inflamed bump, but this one does not have visible pus in the top of it.

Cysts, zits, bumps. These are larger, deeper, tender lesions. Often they are so deep in the skin that they may never come to a head, never develop visible pus. These are the ones that are most likely to leave scars.

So, from the dermatologist's perspective, just about any kind of small or large bump, whether few or many, constitutes a verdict of acne. That's the way it is; do not be insulted if someone says you have acne. Just read on to learn more about acne and what you can do about it.

CAUSES

Blackheads, whiteheads, pimples, pustules, and cysts all probably spring from the same fundamental causes. There are three basic parts to the cause of acne:

1. Active oil glands. By definition, acne is a disorder of active oil glands. The activity of oil glands is determined by heredity and hormones.
2. Blocking or plugging of oil ducts and pores. The small channel through which oil gets to the skin surface may become blocked by a mixture of dead skin cells and oil. Acne problems do not often occur on skin areas where pores are visibly large. That is probably because of a large pore just does not get blocked easily. *Acne very often occurs on the chin area of women past teenage,* probably because the oil glands are big there but the pores are very small, and therefore easily blocked.
3. Bacteria normally present on everyone's skin may enter the blocked pore and cause it to develop into a pimple, pustule, or cyst.

So now that you know that those breakouts are called acne, that a large number of mature women have acne, and about some of the basic definitions of acne lesions; read on to learn about the various factors that predispose to acne, and may be involved in your own case. Then action can be taken to correct the problem. The last part of this section is about what can be done on your own about the problem—about skin-care routines and medications for acne—and what dermatologists can do.

Acne Means Oily Skin

Acne is, by definition, a disorder of active oil glands. It has been proven scientifically that acne occurs only in individuals who have fairly high oil-secretion levels. Just remember: *Acne means oily skin in the areas where the acne problem is.*

A Changing Skin at Age Thirty

Many women undergo a significant skin change sometime between ages twenty-five and thirty-five. This is a change in oil glands, toward bigger, more active oil glands—toward oilier and therefore more acne-prone skin.

Women have been told for so long that their skins are drying out at age thirty that they have a difficult time believing they could possibly be getting oilier at this time. Though not well documented scientifically, this change toward oilier skin is very often noted by dermatologists. Some signs of this change toward oilier skin:

> *Pores become larger*—and we know that big pores mean big oil glands.
>
> *Seborrheic dermatitis develops* in the scalp (dandruff and itching) and on the face. These problems, though often interpreted as dry scalp and dry skin, are really a result of oily skin. There is more about seborrheic dermatitis in chapter 15.
>
> *Acne breakout problems often develop* at about age thirty. That should be the most compelling argument yet. For, again, it is a fact that acne occurs only in oily skin.

There is no consensus on what may be causing this change toward more active oil glands. It is logical to postulate that changing hormone patterns are the cause. Small changes in the relative amounts of male and female hormones can cause large changes in oil glands.

Birth-Control Pills and Breakout Problems

There are lots of birth-control pills on the market, and they contain different hormones, at different dose levels. Their effect—good or bad—on acne problems depends not only on what the pill contains but on the hormone and oil gland complexities of the woman taking the pill. Acne breakout problems may improve or worsen when birth-control pills are started. Some types of birth-control pill usually help an acne problem; other types may, in susceptible individuals, aggravate or even cause an acne problem.

Birth-control pills contain two hormones—an estrogen and a progesterone. Those pills containing a relatively high dose of estrogen are usually better at controlling acne than those with a low estrogen dose. Those higher-dose pills also cause more of the usual pill side effects.

For the acne-prone patient the type of progestin hormone is important—norethinodrone and norgestrel have some male-hormone-like activity, and pills containing it are usually *not* recommended by dermatologists for the acne-prone woman. Birth-control pills containing ethynodiol diacetate as the progestin seem to be better at helping the faces of acne-prone women, because that type of progestin does not have significant male-hormone activity.

Starting birth-control pills. When a woman begins taking birth-control pills that are the wrong kind for her, her face may break out quickly—in a matter of weeks. When the right kind of pill is started, she usually will not break out at all. But if the pill is being taken to help a preexisting case of acne, she probably will not notice improvement for a long time—three or four months. It takes that long to modulate hormone levels.

Stopping birth-control pills. Most of the breakout problems associated with birth-control pills seem to happen upon stopping the pill. The reason for this is that while a woman is on the pill, her natural hormones have been suppressed; when the pills are stopped, the natural hormones start up again, and often seem to be "out of balance." Until the natural hormones have settled back to normal (which may take several months), acne problems may be a real bother.

Hormone Problems and Acne

Recent scientific studies are shedding more light on the problem of acne in women past teen age. Although these studies do not all seem to agree with each other, the general truth that comes from them is that a significant percentage of women who have acne past teen age do have hormone abnormalities—higher than normal levels of male-type hormones. These levels are almost never high enough to cause obvious masculine changes but are high enough to cause acne. These women are "normal" enough in the hormone department to have normal female hair patterns, to have regular menstrual periods, and to be fertile.

A very few women, though, do have hormone levels so far from normal that they show obvious physical changes in addition to acne: excessive hair growth in typical male areas such as the beard region (even male-type baldness can appear), absence or abnormalities of menstrual periods, and infertility. Women in this category must definitely be under the care of a physician—endocrinologists and gynecologists are specialists in this area—as these may be signs of serious physical problems.

What tests can be done? When abnormalities of hormones are suspected, appropriate testing can be done to determine the problem. Gynecologists, dermatologists, and other physicians can have these tests done for you. They have only recently become generally available. These are blood tests for male hormone levels and they are expensive.

New facts are being discovered in this area each year. You must rely upon a physician expert in this area to help guide you about whether hormone tests and hormone treatments are appropriate for you.

Cosmetics and Acne

Cleansers, moisturizers, bases, foundations, blushers, and even sun-screening lotions may cause previously clear skin to break out; all may make a very minor acne problem into a major one. It is a fact that the wrong cosmetic and skin-care products used on acne-prone skin can cause or worsen acne. Dermatologists call this problem "acne cosmetica" and see it every day. The constant call to moisturize, moisturize, moisturize is responsible for a lot of pimples! One of the most important messages in this book: *Do not moisturize acne-prone areas of the face.* Do not use moisturizing foundations, moisturizing blushers, or anything else moisturizing on acne-prone areas of the face. Fortunately, at least a few cosmetic makers are finally coming around to understand this problem and are providing better cosmetic and skin-care products for acne-prone women.

The problem of just how cosmetics promote acne is complicated. Dermatologists and cosmetic manufacturers alike are far from understanding it completely. Tests have been devised to try to determine whether a cosmetic ingredient or formula is likely to cause acne problems. Lists of particularly offensive chemicals are available; at least some, if not most, cosmetic manufacturers avoid using them.

Some cosmetic manufacturers are becoming more aware of this problem and are searching for noncomedogenic cosmetic and skin-care formulas. "Noncomedogenic" means that a chemical or mixture does not cause comedones (blackheads) when applied to skin in laboratory tests. Currently the inside of the rabbit ear is the most used test area. Research is in progress to find a better way to test for the comedogenicity or acne-causing potential of a cosmetic product.

But, unfortunately, the tests for comedogenicity are not good enough yet—products that pass the tests still cause breakout problems on some faces. As of the time of this writing, a label or advertising claim of "noncomedogenic" does not guarantee safety. But it does at least mean that the maker of that product is trying. There is more on this subject in chapter 7.

The most comedogenic products put on very acne-prone faces can cause noticeable problems quickly—within weeks; relatively less offensive products put on slightly acne-prone faces may not cause problems until the product has been used for three to six months. And there are all degrees between these two extremes. Therefore, it is difficult sometimes to decide if cosmetic products are causing problems at all. But the truth is that they often are. The problem is further compounded by the fact that women in general are using more cosmetic products that ever before, and most women around age thirty are using more cosmetic products than when they were younger. There are more imperfections to cover up. They see little facial lines and are convinced by beautiful cosmetic ads and incorrect skin-care advice that they need more and more moisturizing products.

Important: *Do not moisturize acne-prone areas of the face.* This applies to the use of moisturizers and moisturizing makeup foundations. Even if they are labeled "noncomedogenic," they may not be safe.

There is more on specific recommendations for skin-care products and cosmetics for the acne-prone face in chapters 11 and 12.

Other Factors That Cause Acne

Acne is such a common problem in the teenage years and beyond, that it has to be considered simply normal. Most individuals who have acne breakout problems are never able to ascertain a specific cause, such as hormone imbalance, birth-control pills, improper cosmetic and skin-care practices, etc. Having acne breakouts may just be the way it is for an individual's skin.

Here are some other factors that seem to cause acne breakouts, or at least aggravate acne:

Heat and humidity.

Exercise, with the resulting perspiration.

Premenstrual hormone changes.

Stress, with the resulting hormone changes.

Diet. So much has been written and discussed about dietary influences on acne! Frankly, there has never been much presented in the way of proof of any of it. Chocolate, coffee, cola, nuts, butterfat, greasy foods, rich foods, foods high in iodine—all of these and more have been implicated in acne. The best approach is to understand that there are wide variations among individuals. Those who feel or know for sure that certain food substances aggravate their acne problems should simply avoid those things.

TREATING THE ACNE BREAKOUTS

If hormones or birth-control pill problems are suspected as the cause, a physician should be consulted and testing done if appropriate. Dermatologists, gynecologists, and endocrinologists all share expertise in this area.

If the acne problem is not so severe, home treatment may suffice, using good medications available without a doctor's prescription. More severe or unresponsive cases should definitely be under the care of a dermatologist.

But, whether treatment for acne is being done at home with nonprescription medications or under a dermatologist's supervision, the proper understanding of and approach to treatment is essential.

Acne medications, prescription or nonprescription, do several things:

Dry and clear pimples.

Kill the germs that are waiting to cause new pimples.

Unblock (by their peeling action) blocked pores.

Prevent blocking of pores.

Prevent acne breakout.

Acne Cleansers

Soaps that contain sulfur and salicylic acid. These are nonprescription items that help acne by their drying and peeling action.

Soaps and liquid cleansers that contain benzoyl peroxide. There are prescription-only and nonprescription products available. They help by their drying, peeling action, and they also kill skin germs.

Cleansers that contain granules. These contain just granules and "soap," or may contain sulfur, salicylic acid, or benzoyl peroxide. They are strong and are appropriate only for very oily, nonsensitive facial skins.

Alcohol-based acne cleansers. These contain alcohol and sometimes other solvents and chemicals. They remove oil, dead skin cells, and germs. They are fine to use, but some can be too drying on sensitive skin.

Acne Medications

Benzoyl peroxide lotion and gels. These are the choice of most dermatologists. They kill germs, and the stronger ones cause beneficial drying and peeling. There are prescription-only and nonprescription products available. They come in strengths from 2.5 to 10 percent. There are tinted products (good for covering and spot-treating a bump) and products that dry clear (best for use over the whole acne-prone area—and you must use medications that way if you want to prevent new bumps). They can bleach any colored fabric they touch, and can cause allergic reactions in some individuals.

Sulfur (and salicylic acid or resorcinol) lotions and gels. These medications are fine to use but in general are not as effective as benzoyl peroxide medications. They are especially useful for individuals allergic to benzoyl peroxide. They are available as tinted or clear products. The tinted ones are good for covering and drying an acne bump.

Retinoic acid medications, Retin A. These are prescription-only products and must be prescribed by your doctor. These medications are used as the mainstay of acne treatment by some dermatologists.

Antibiotic lotions and creams. These are also prescription-only products. They are recommended by many dermatologists.

Acne masks. Two products, Neutrogena Acne Mask and Vlemasque (both available without prescription), are often recommended by dermatologists. They do a nice job of medicating and cleansing. They can be a part of nearly every acne-control program.

Antibiotic capsules and tablets. These drugs are of immense value in treating acne. Tetracycline, minocycline, and erythromycin are the primary ones prescribed. Some seem quite safe for long-term use, some not so safe. Some are quite expensive, some quite *inexpensive*. Let your dermatologist guide you in the appropriate use of these prescription drugs.

13 Cis-retinoic acid, Accutane. This powerful medication is relatively new and is truly a wonder drug for severe acne. It is expensive and has side effects, but it is so effective that it should be considered by anyone with severe or otherwise unresponsive acne problems. In some cases it permanently cures the acne tendency. It must not (absolutely not) be taken if there is a chance of becoming pregnant while taking it, for there is a very high risk of damage to the developing fetus. Severe birth defects may result.

Zinc. Zinc supplements have been said to help acne in some cases, though convincing evidence is lacking. Ask your dermatologist about this, and do not take zinc without a doctor's supervision.

Vitamins A and E. There is no question that vitamin A is helpful in some cases of acne. Its effect is enhanced if it is taken along with vitamin E. The problem, though, is that the dose of vitamin A required to really help acne is fairly high. Taking high doses of vitamin A, or even moderate doses for too long, is risky, for toxic effects can be severe. Like 13 Cis-retinoic acid, vitamin A can cause birth defects. Do not take these vitamins for acne without specific instructions from your dermatologist.

ACNE TREATMENT—DAILY ROUTINES

If your facial skin is troubled by occasional or constant outbreaks, start doing something about it now. Use available nonprescription medications *on a regular daily basis,* or consult a dermatologist and use the prescribed medications on a *regular daily basis.* It is ever so important to remember that *daily treatment is the key* in preventing any type of acne outbreak.

Cleansing—night and morning. Use fairly strong cleansing measures: medicated cleansers if your skin is not too sensitive, and scrubbing cleansers or scrubbing grains or pads if your skin is very oily and not sensitive. *Never* scrub hard. Use warm water, not hot. Use cleansing masks such as Vlemasque or Neutrogena Acne Mask, and astringents or fresheners, if you like. Never fail to use a lathering cleanser even if your skin is sensitive. Mild ones are available. (See "Acne Products," page 124.)

Moisturizing. It is risky to moisturize acne-prone skin areas. It may be better to tolerate a little surface dryness in the effort to avoid pimples. Even the so-called oil-free and noncomedogenic moisturizers are not entirely safe. When women really learn this, they will not spend as much time and money at the dermatologist's office! See chapter 11.

Medicating. You should always medicate overnight and morning and night if you can. Start with a relatively mild acne medication (benzoyl peroxide preferred), and then increase the strength of the acne medication as your skin can tolerate it. A little drying and peeling is needed for good effect. Medicate every day, even if your face is clear—this helps *prevent* new outbreaks. (See "Acne Products," below.)

Cosmetics. Please reread chapter 12—the part that discusses makeup for acne-prone skin.

ACNE PRODUCTS

CLEANSERS
Nonmedicated
Purpose Soap
Acne Aid Bar
Neutrogena for Oily Skin
Phisoderm (liquid and bar)
pHresh 3.5 (liquid)
Aveenobar (for acne)
Almay Oil Control Cleansing Lotion

Medicated
(BP: with benzoyl peroxide)
Fostex Medicated Cleansing Bar
Fostex 10% BP Cleansing Bar (BP)
Oxy Clean Soap
Oxy Wash (BP)
Sastid Soap

SCRUB CLEANSERS
Oxy Clean Scrub (BP)
Pernox Medicated Scrub Cleanser

MEDICATIONS
Benzoyl Peroxide types
Oxy 5% and 10% (dries clear)
Clear by Design 2.5% (dries clear)

Benoxyl 5% and 10% (dries clear)
Persadox 5% and 10% (dries clear)
Dry & Clear 5% and 10% (dries clear)
Fostex 10% (BP) (dries clear)
Noxzema Acne 12 (dries clear)
Clearasil Vanishing Formula (dries clear)
Oxy 10 Cover (tinted)
Clearasil Tinted Formula
Vanoxide (tinted)

Sulfur Types
Transact Gel (dries clear)
Xerac Gel (dries clear)
Phiso-AC (dries clear)
Propa PH (dries clear)
Rezamid (tinted)
Acnomel Acne Cream (tinted)
Clearasil Adult Care (tinted)

BLEMISH-SPOT COVERUP, MEDICATED
Almay Touch on Blemish Treatment
Noxzema on the Spot (10% BP)
Clinique Touch-Stick Lotion
Clearasil Regular Tinted Stick
Janet Sartin Blemish Fix
Germaine Monteil Medicated Cover Up Treatment

THE APPROACH TO ACNE TREATMENT

Acne medications should be applied to the entire skin area that is acne-prone, not just to acne bumps. Acne medications *do* help make bumps clear up more quickly; more important, they are being used to prevent new bumps.

Acne medications must be used every day. Acne medications do help prevent bumps. Logically, this means that the patient should continue to use them even when the skin is clear, to help keep it clear. It simply does not make sense to get the skin cleared up, then stop medicating until another crop of bumps appears.

Persistence and patience are required. To achieve good results, an acne patient must treat the problem consistently, daily, for a long time. It may take two or three months of daily treatment to see a really significant change in an acne problem. Good results may be seen sooner, but this should not be expected.

HOW TO TAKE THE OFFENSIVE AGAINST MONTHLY BREAKOUTS

Keeping track of your face's breakout pattern for a few months can help you take the offensive against skin troubles. Whether you break out premenstrually or before ovulation, you'll most likely stick to that same pattern month after month (so long as you don't go on or off the pill). So a few days before you usually break out, you can switch to a stronger cleanser and apply a lighter moisturizer (or none at all in acne-prone spots) and dab an anti-acne medication (benzoyl peroxide or any of the other acne medications listed in this chapter) on known trouble spots. Since benzoyl peroxide (and others) nips acne-causing bacteria before they can cause a pimple to bloom, you should experience fewer, less extensive breakouts as the months pass.

SPOT CLEARING—FOR THAT BIG RED BUMP

The average pimple lasts about a week in its full-blown red glory, but you can shorten its stay to a few days with the following quick-clearing regimen.

The moment you see or feel a pimple coming on, apply a drying agent just before you go to bed. The most effective choices are either a 10 percent benzoyl peroxide solution or a medicated acne mask (such as Dermik Laboratories Vlemasque or Neutrogena Acne Mask). In a pinch, calamine lotion will do—it dries and absorbs excess oil. Apply these only to newly washed skin—surface oil may hinder the product's effectiveness. If the bump seems really red or swollen, try applying an ice cube to it for one to two minutes—cold reduces inflammation—then applying the drying agent. The following morning, cover the blemish with tinted acne coverup, such as Clinique Anti-Acne Control, Shiseido Pureness Spot Cream, or Clearasil Tinted Cream. Repeat this process daily until the bump clears.

Important Comments and Cautions

Most acne medications cause some drying and perhaps slight peeling of the skin surface. This means that the medication is strong enough to do some good. The drying effect does not have to be severe to be helpful—just a slight "chapped" condition is the level of dryness needed. This drying effect is absolutely *not* harmful to skin. It will not produce wrinkles or any other harm to the skin.

One caution here: Brown- or black-skinned individuals should avoid extreme dryness from acne medications, as darkening of the treated skin areas may result.

Dryness from acne medications should not be counteracted by the use of moisturizers. Resist the urge if you want to stop having breakouts. Even "oil-free" or "noncomedogenic" moisturizers are not safe for acne-prone skin. Some facial areas are more sensitive than others. If those areas get too dry, do not treat them as often; continue the daily treatment of other areas.

The degree of dryness from acne medications will depend upon the strength of the medication, the frequency of use, your skin type, and the climate and humidity. Low-humidity climates and sensitive skin dictate mild medicines. Use common sense in your selection.

If an acne medication causes significant itching, swelling, or blistering of the face, you may have become allergic to something in it. Benzoyl peroxide is the most common cause of allergic reactions, but other types of medications can cause reactions, too. Fortunately, these reactions are fairly rare. Allergic reactions to acne medication can be easily taken care of by stopping all medicated products and applying, several times daily, a .5 percent hydrocortisone cream, which is available without a doctor's prescription. Your dermatologist can prescribe more powerful medications for even quicker clearing. When the allergic reaction has completely cleared, select a chemically different type of acne medication and proceed.

SEBORRHEIC DERMATITIS

15

Seborrheic dermatitis is second only to acne in the list of common facial problems, and is certainly the most misunderstood of all.

WHAT IS IT?

Let's take the name apart: "Seborrheic" is an adjective that simply means "oily." "Dermatitis" is a noun that means "irritated skin." The irritation shows up as red, scaly, flaky, and maybe itchy skin. So seborrheic dermatitis is a dermatitis of oily skin areas. Since the face and scalp both contain lots of oil glands, they are the prime sites of seborrheic dermatitis. Yet seborrheic dermatitis is usually mistaken for dry skin. Almost everyone who has seborrheic dermatitis is sure that it is dry skin, for it always produces flaking and scaling.

Seborrheic dermatitis is often mistaken for "combination skin," which is usually defined as a face that has dry areas and oily areas.

It is no wonder individuals almost always think that seborrheic dermatitis is dry skin or combination skin, for those who sell cosmetics and give skin-care advice almost always fail to recognize seborrheic dermatitis. The constantly repeated, erroneous "analysis" and bad advice is that you have *very* dry skin that need *lots* of moisturizers—the heavier the better!

The prime locations of seborrheic dermatitis are the hairline, especially the front and sides; the brows and forehead; the eyelids, and sometimes the eyelashes; the skin at the sides of the nose; above and behind the ears, and in the ear canals; in any facial crease; and the scalp—especially "dry," itchy, dandruffy ones.

In appearance seborrheic dermatitis is like any other mild dermatitis—red, scaly (or maybe just slightly rough-feeling), and itchy (maybe just a little bit).

128

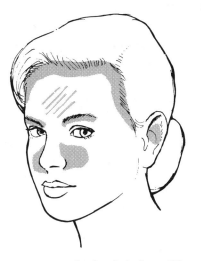

The pattern of seborrheic dermatitis.

It is especially important to note that seborrheic dermatitis of the face is almost always accompanied by seborrheic dermatitis of the scalp. The scalp problem is perceived as "dry scalp," itching, or dandruff. Those who think they have dry scalp (the hairdresser told them) will usually admit that their hair gets oily or "dirty" quickly, and they need to shampoo often. This indicates that they have very active scalp oil glands, and therefore the scalp is not "dry."

The point of all this is that scalp problems are often the big clue to the diagnosis of facial dermatitis as seborrheic dermatitis.

THE CAUSE OF SEBORRHEIC DERMATITIS

Not much is known about this condition, but a reasonable theory is that microbes normally present on everyone's skin are the culprits. The microbes feed on skin oils and, when fed too well, run rampant and cause the dermatitis. They are present on everyone but cause trouble only for those who have oily facial skin and scalp, and only in those areas of extra oiliness. Since not every person with oily skin has seborrheic dermatitis, the chemical composition of an individual's oil secretions may play a role.

Also, some individuals tend to flake and scale more easily than others. That is because the top thin layer of skin, the stratum corneum, varies in its thickness, flexibility, moisture-holding abilities, and general integrity. Those who have a stratum corneum that dries and flakes easily, and who have big, active oil glands, get seborrheic dermatitis much more often and more severely. Indeed, it is quite the normal thing for individuals with facial seborrheic dermatitis to have considerable trouble with flaky skin elsewhere on the body—hands, legs, etc.

Seborrheic dermatitis may develop at almost any age. When infants get it, it's called "cradle cap." They have it because maternal hormones give them oily scalps for the first few months of life.

Another prime time for development of seborrheic dermatitis is in early teenage years, at the beginning of puberty, when increasing hormone levels cause greatly increased facial and scalp oil flow. The usual area of involvement at this age is the skin beside the nose. It may show up before acne problems do.

Twenty-five- to thirty-five-year-old women seem to be affected often. The cause here is probably another hormone change—one that often also causes a time of acne breakouts. In this group, inadequate skin cleansing and too much moisturizing are provoking factors.

And finally, from fifty years on is another prime time for seborrheic dermatitis, both in men and women.

Ups and Downs

At whatever age you have it, seborrheic dermatitis tends to wax and wane. Once it develops, its victims always seem prone to have it again and again. Treatments do not *cure* it but can very effectively *control* it.

FACTORS THAT MAKE SEBORRHEIC DERMATITIS WORSE
Cold weather and low humidity
Absence of sun exposure
Poor cleansing of face and scalp
Stress

FACTORS THAT MAKE SEBORRHEIC DERMATITIS BETTER
Warm, humid weather—humidity makes facial skin less apt to flake.
Sunlight—though it may seem to worsen the problem at first.
Thorough cleansing of facial skin—it removes oil, scales, and the microbes that cause the problem.
Proper scalp care—it is almost always necessary to control scalp problems to control facial problems.

TREATMENT

Seborrheic dermatitis is a problem you can usually take care of yourself with proper cleansing, shampooing, and medicating. In dealing with seborrheic dermatitis, remember that you will not permanently cure the problem, but you can adequately control it. When you get better, do not stop your efforts completely. Treat yourself intensively to get the problem under control, then less intensively to keep it that way.

Cleansing is important. Good cleansing removes oil, dead skin cells (which you perceive as flakes,) and the microbes that cause the problem. Cleansing does not have to be fancy, just thorough and gentle. See chapter 9 and follow the guidelines there. The most important thing is to use a lathering cleanser. Only lathering cleansers can really float those microbes up and off the skin and down the drain.

Shampooing frequently with "medicated" shampoos. This is almost always necessary in order to help control facial seborrheic dermatitis— whether or not you think you have a scalp problem. Shampoo often— once a week is just not enough. Three to five times weekly is much better. Use medicated shampoos if the frequent use of nonmedicated ones is not doing the job. Many gentle and effective products are now available. (See the table at the end of this chapter.)

Leave medicated-shampoo lather on the hair for five minutes. It takes that long for these shampoos to work. And alternating shampoo types (see the table) is more effective than staying with the same type all the time.

Conditioners are fine to use.

Moisturizing (a little) helps most mild cases of facial seborrheic dermatitis. Coupled with really good cleansing, moisturizing may be adequate to control the mildest cases of seborrheic dermatitis. But be sure to use a light moisturizing product—never one that leaves the skin feeling oily or greasy. Do not overdo. Too much moisturizing coupled with inadequate cleansing makes seborrheic dermatitis worse.

Medicating is necessary to control most cases of seborrheic dermatitis. A variety of good medications are available over the counter. See the table at the end of this chapter for some suggestions. Pick one that suits you and apply it very sparingly to the involved areas of your face, *twice daily until you are better* and then only as needed to keep it that way. But before plunging into medicating yourself, read this:

Caution about cortisone medications. Those available without a doctor's prescription (.5 percent hydrocortisone) are pretty safe, even for relatively prolonged use. Good advice is to use them no more than twice daily for two to three weeks, then less often. You can't go wrong by following the package instructions; these products can cause skin problems if overused. With this limited facial use, absorption of cortisone into the body is not a concern.

Other cortisone medications. Those available only on prescription can cause even more serious problems if overused, so be cautious with them. Prescription cortisone medications really help get seborrheic dermatitis under control in a hurry—and it is fine to use them twice daily for one week for that purpose—but you must not use them on a regular daily basis. These medications can, with prolonged use, cause permanent thinning of the skin, dilation of facial blood vessels, and some difficult pustular eruptions such as rosacea and severe acne.

Caution about eyelids. Some of the medications listed below are not appropriate for treating seborrheic dermatitis of the eyelids. For help with treating eyelid problems, see chapter 17.

MEDICATIONS

.5 Percent Hydrocortisone Products

Always use the creamy type, not the heavy ointment (like Vaseline) type. Although there are many others, below is a list of some hydrocortisone creams:

> Cortaid cream
> Caldecort cream
> Dermolate cream
> Lanacort cream

Coal Tar Products

The milder ones are pleasant to use. The stronger ones smell and may irritate. Any tar product may occasionally cause allergic skin reactions where you apply them. If this happens to you, stay away from this category.

> Aquatar lotion.
> DOAK Tar lotion.
> Tegrin cream and lotion.

Pragmatar cream—effective for stubborn cases but may irritate. Dilute it half-and-half with a light moisturizing cream or lotion.

Iodochlorhydroxyquin.

Vioform cream. This product stains fabrics yellow; careful and sparing use is a must. This product works even better if mixed half-and-half with hydrocortisone cream.

Miconazole nitrate.

Micatin cream. Sold as an antifungal medication (for athlete's foot, etc.), it also kills the microbes in seborrheic dermatitis. Full strength, it may be irritating. For best results, mix it half-and-half with hydrocortisone cream.

Shampoos for Seborrheic Dermatitis

COAL TAR TYPE (*means mild)
Denorex
Ionil T and Ionil T Plus*
Sebutone
T/gel*
Tegrin

Note: Coal tar shampoos can stain gray, blond, or bleached hair. Read the label and use caution.

SALICYLIC ACID TYPE
Ionil and Ionil Plus
Meted
Sebulex
Vanseb

SELENIUM SULFIDE TYPE
Selsun Blue

ZINC PYRITHIONE TYPE
Danex
Head and Shoulders
Sebulon
Zincon

There are other shampoos of each of these types available. Read the label to learn which active ingredient each contains.

16

ADVERSE REACTIONS TO COSMETICS

The kinds of reactions to cosmetics we are discussing here are the allergic or irritant ones. Breaking out with acne bumps is another subject altogether and is covered in chapter 14.

Dermatologists hear about and read about facial cosmetic and skin-care product "allergic" reactions but do not actually see them often. Reactions from hair products—dyes, permanent wave solutions, mousses, pomades, etc.—are pretty common. Those reactions do affect facial skin, especially at ears and hairline. But reactions from *facial* cosmetic and skin-care products are fairly rare in the dermatologist's office. Considering the very many skin-care products that are used and the minor nature of most of these reactions, the incidence of serious reactions is really pretty low. This is a real credit to the skin-care industry, which produces pure, high-quality, and well-tested products for the consumer. The industry certainly does not want adverse reactions to products, so they try hard to market only those that pass rigorous tests. A bad product does occasionally get marketed; it is usually withdrawn quickly when it causes trouble.

Just for the fun of it, lay out all the skin-care and cosmetic products you use: cleansers, astringent, makeup remover, eye makeup remover, mask, lipstick, foundation, powder, perfume, eye shadow, eye liner, blush, hair spray, shampoo, conditioner (are there more?). Now write down (or at least count) the chemical ingredients of each of the products. How many did you come up with? Fifty, eighty, one hundred fifty? Is it any real wonder that allergic and irritant reactions occur?

HYPOALLERGENIC COSMETICS

The word "hypoallergenic" is much used and much misunderstood by the public. Most consumers have taken it to mean non-allergenic, but that just isn't true.

In general terms, "hypoallergenic" means "does not cause *many* allergic reactions."

There is no FDA-regulatory definition of "hypoallergenic," nor is there a standard across the cosmetic industry. There is no single standard by which to decide whether a product is hypoallergenic. So, unfortunately, the term has little real meaning.

The fact is that most brand-name cosmetic and skin-care products are safe and do not cause many allergic reactions, and, thus, are "hypoallergenic" in practice.

The label "hypoallergenic" does *not* mean that a cosmetic product so labeled cannot cause a reaction on your skin, only that it does not cause problems for many individuals. Your allergies and sensitivities are your own and highly individualized. Just because a cosmetic product does not often cause problems in other people does not mean that it is guaranteed safe for you.

DIAGNOSING COSMETIC REACTIONS

It is usually easy—you use a cosmetic product, often for the first time, and a day or a week or a month later an itchy rash occurs where this product is being put on the skin. You stop using that product, change to a different brand or type, and the reaction clears up and stays clear. That scenario accounts for the statement made earlier that dermatologists do not encounter very many cosmetic reactions—the individual made a common-sense diagnosis and did not need professional help. Most women have the intelligence and common sense to figure out what caused the problem and seek the obvious solution: change.

But figuring out cosmetic reactions is sometimes far more difficult, even for a skilled dermatologist. If the cause of a cosmetic reaction is not immediatley obvious and you want to be your own detective, here are some pointers.

Fragrances, scents, and preservatives are the most common offenders. Use unscented and fragrance-free cosmetic products (see chapter 7). The preservatives in question are usually the parabens (methyl butyl and propyl paraben), but there are many other preservatives, and new ones are being added all the time. Many of them have caused allergic sensitivity. Imidazolidinyl urea, DM and DMDM hydantoin, Quarternium 15, and Kathon CG are some of the difficult chemical names you may see at the bottom of the ingredients list. If you want to know which chemical in your skin-care product is the preservative, the last name on the ingredients list is almost surely it.

If you are sensitive to fragrances or scents, be wary in your use of so-called botanicals—plant extracts. Botanical ingredients may sound soothing and natural but can cause reactions in those sensitive to fragrances.

Propylene glycol, another common cosmetic ingredient, also causes some problems. Sensitive skins should not use cosmetics containing propylene glycol—especially if it is close to the top on the list of ingredients (that means there is a lot of it in the product.)

A cosmetic or skin-care product may cause a reaction on your skin even if you have been using it for months or years with no trouble. It may be that it just took that long for you to develop sensitivity to it, *or* a product's ingredients were changed without your knowing it.

Hair products—shampoos, conditioners, and sprays—do get on the facial skin and may be causing the problem. Try to avoid facial contact with these products. Hold a towel over the face when using hair spray; keep the head tilted back when shampooing and conditioning.

Eyelid skin is very thin and sensitive. Eyelid skin may react to any product used on the face—cleansers, foundation, perfume, powder— even if not specifically used on the eyelids. Stroking an itchy eyelid with polished nails may produce a nail polish allergy on the eyelid.

TESTING FOR COSMETIC REACTIONS

A test you can do to straighten out a confused picture of facial cosmetic reactions is the "use test." Outline one-inch squares on the inside of your forearm—one for each of your facial skin-care and cosmetic products. Apply, twice daily, each product to its own square. Do this for five days. If one of your products is a troublemaker, you should get red and itchy in the square you are putting it on. But nothing is perfect; a product may irritate facial skin and not irritate arm skin.

A trial-and-error process for determining the offending agent is to stop using *all* cosmetic and skin-care products, treat if necessary (as discussed below), and wait a few days until all signs of the reactions are gone. Then, one at a time, start using your products, giving each a few days to react before adding the next one. Do not do this if the reaction you had was a severe one; a use test on your arm is more sensible. In this way you should be able to determine the offending product.

TREATING COSMETIC REACTIONS

For severe reactions—redness, swelling, and itching—stop all cosmetic and skin-care products and see your dermatologist without delay.

For mild reactions—just a little redness and itching—you may want to try nonprescription medications, such as .5 percent hydrocortisone cream, which is the medicine of choice. Pick up a tube in your nearest pharmacy—it is available without prescription. Apply it thinly but thoroughly four times daily.

And of course, while you are treating a cosmetic reaction, do not use any cosmetic or skin-care products until the rash has cleared, and you have decided which product caused the problem.

Cosmetic and Skin Care for Allergic or Sensitive Skin

First, keep it simple. The fewer products used means the fewer possible chemicals to cause you problems. And use simpler products—the ones with the fewest ingredients on the list.

Second, use products labeled "unscented," "fragrance-free," and "hypoallergenic." Those labels do not guarantee that your skin will tolerate these products, but they are helpful. Ask your dermatologist for the names of products that in his or her experience cause the fewest problems.

THE PROBLEM OF SUPERSENSITIVE SKIN

There are individuals (fortunately, not many) whose facial skin cannot seem to tolerate anything. Any cosmetic product causes itching, stinging, and redness. This situation has been called "status cosmeticus," and those affected have been nicknamed "stingers."

The situation can be a baffling one, and a solution is often difficult to find. A dermatologist's counsel should be sought. You may have an underlying dermatitis such as seborrheic or atopic dermatitis, which will require treatment before your skin will ever settle down.

Here are some measures you can try on your own:

Cleanse the face with warm water *only.*

Apply .5 percent hydrocortisone ointment. (That is the kind that is like Vaseline in consistency—ask your pharmacist for it.) Apply it twice daily, sparingly, until the skin settles down (is no longer irritated). Prolonged use of over-the-counter hydrocortisone can be harmful to facial skin, but these products can be safely used twice daily for two weeks, then from time to time as needed.

Most of the time, just do not use other skin-care or cosmetic products. Perhaps eye makeup, loose powder, and powder blush will be tolerated and give you a little color. When you just have to be more "made-up" than that, add a foundation—a simple, light one that contains *no propylene glycol,* is labeled "hypoallergenic," and is both unscented and fragrance-free.

EYELID DERMATITIS

17

The thin and sensitive skin of the eyelids seems to get itchy and flaky at the slightest provocation. That's because eyelid skin is the thinnest and most sensitive skin of the entire body.

When eyelid dermatitis strikes, it is usually just a little red, flaky, itchy bother, but it can be more severe, with swelling and even splitting of the tender eyelid skin. When it strikes you, this chapter will help you decide why it happened and what you can do about it.

Anyone can develop eyelid dermatitis, but the problem is far more likely in individuals who:

Have seborrheic dermatitis (see chapter 15)
Have, or have a history of, asthma, hay fever, or allergic (atopic) eczema
Are occupationally exposed to irritating chemicals
Have become allergic to cosmetic and skin-care products

THE CAUSES OF EYELID DERMATITIS

No matter what the cause of eyelid dermatitis, it all looks pretty much the same, so you cannot rely on the *appearance* of eyelid dermatitis to help you much in determining the cause. The following is a discussion of the various causes of the problem. After reading it, you will have a better idea of what caused your eyelid dermatitis.

Seborrheic Dermatitis

If you have eyelid dermatitis and seborrheic dermatitis, seborrheic dermatitis is almost surely the cause of the eyelid dermatitis. Seborrheic dermatitis is manifested by flaking and itching of the scalp (dandruff), ears, brows, and cheeks at the sides of the nose. Since seborrheic dermatitis is the leading cause of eyelid dermatitis, it should be thoroughly understood by all who have eyelid dermatitis. Read chapter 15 before going on.

Seborrheic dermatitis may be the *primary* cause of eyelid dermatitis, or it may be a *contributing* cause. The tendency to seborrheic dermatitis may set the scene for irritation from cosmetic and skin-care products.

Allergies and Eczema

Individuals who have a tendency to, or history of, respiratory allergies such as asthma and hay fever, and of allergic or atopic eczema, are more prone to eyelid dermatitis.

Pollens and other airborne allergies seem to play a role in eyelid dermatitis in this group. Spring and fall (the high allergy seasons) are when most eyelid dermatitis shows up at the dermatologist's office.

The other factor in this allergic group is that they just seem to have more sensitive skin than normal, more apt to be irritated by, or allergic to, cosmetic and skin-care ingredients. Also, they have skin allergic to any other chemical substances that get on the lids.

Allergies and Sensitivities to Chemicals

At home or at work, there may be chemicals that can cause eyelid dermatitis. Eyelid skin is so thin and sensitive that it may react when no other skin area does. Chemicals that produce fumes may cause problems by being in the air at home or at work. Chemicals that get on the hands are easily transferred to the eyelids by touching and rubbing.

At home, suspect any cleaning product, wax, and all hobby chemicals—glue, paint, solvents, and sawdust.

At the office, suspect any chemically treated paper and copying chemicals.

At the plant, suspect airborne fumes and any other solvents or chemicals with which you are working.

Contact lens wearers should suspect the preservative (usually thimersol-merthiolate) in any of the lens solutions.

Allergies and Sensitivities to Cosmetic and Skin-Care Products

This topic is discussed last on the list of things that may cause eyelid dermatitis, even though it is usually the first cause that comes to mind. Many dermatologists feel that sensitivity to cosmetic and skin-care products is not the most common cause of eyelid dermatitis.

But cosmetic and skin-care products do certainly sometimes cause the problem, either by being the primary culprit—irritating healthy eyelid skin—or just by further aggravating eyelid skin that is already affected by seborrheic dermatitis or atopic (allergic) eczema.

The following products may come into contact with eyelid skin and cause eyelid dermatitis:

Soap and other cleansing products
Eye makeup remover
Moisturizers
Special "eye-line" products
Special cosmetic products like Eye Fix
Foundation
Concealer or cover stick
Eye shadow of various types
Eye liner
Mascara

And a few other things you may not think about:

Shampoo
Conditioner
Hair spray
Bath soap
Perfume—it drifts everywhere
Nail cosmetics—from back-handed stroking of the lids

And all these products contain multiple ingredients—just look at those labels. Is it any wonder that it may sometimes be so difficult to determine the specific sensitivity that caused the eyelid dermatitis?

Eyelid skin may react to products that do not bother other facial skin areas. It is very important to remember about the extreme thinness and sensitivity of eyelid skin when trying to sort out this problem.

Almost any product that contacts eyelid skin may cause the problem. Irritation occurs and allergies develop from "new" products in your skin-care and cosmetic routine, or even from products you have used for a long while. These "old" products may have changed ingredients, or your skin may just have become more sensitive.

It usually takes a while—two weeks or more—to develop a true allergy to a new skin-care product. It only takes a day or two to react (develop dermatitis) to a product or ingredient to which you are already allergic.

WHICH PRODUCT CAUSED THE PROBLEM?

By taking some logical steps, you may be able to find out on your own what is causing your eyelid dermatitis. Here's how:

1. Be sure you have read chapter 15 and have looked at your face, ears, and scalp for signs of that problem.
2. Rule out the possibility that a non-eye product is causing the problem. Be *very* careful to avoid eyelid contact with hair spray, shampoos and conditioners, nail enamel, and fancy or scented bath soaps.
3. *Simplify* eyelid care and cosmetics. Stop using things that are not absolutely necessary, and use the simplest products.

    For example, for removing eye makeup use a little baby shampoo and water (a new product, Occusoft Lid Scrub, is now available for this special purpose); use plain mineral oil first if you need to. Use simple eyelid moisturizers (if you moisturize). Try just a tiny bit of petrolatum (Vaseline). And that's all—simplify!
4. Change eye makeup products. One good change is from "waterproof" cosmetics to ones that are not, or vice versa. Change to hypoallergenic, unscented, fragrance-free products for all your facial cosmetic needs. Change from your present brand of eye cosmetics to another.
5. Discard any old eye makeup products—mascara, shadows, liners, crayons. After a few months, the preservatives in these products break down, and these makeups can become contaminated by microorganisms that can cause dermatitis or an eye infection.

    Microbes, as has been mentioned, are always present on the human body and can be transferred to eye makeup via an applicator, fingers, or saliva. Unfortunately, you may not know your product is contaminated until it is too late. Three ways to protect yourself:

    - Don't buy preservative-free products. (Of course, if you are allergic to a particular preservative, don't buy that product.)
    - Before you apply any eye product, sniff it. If it smells "off" or spoiled, don't apply it.
    - Date your makeup. Note the day and month of purchase on the label, or write it on a self-adhesive label or a strip of masking tape and stick it on the product. The maximum shelf life of eye products is six months.

Usually these maneuvers will, sooner or later, give you an answer to the question of what caused your eyelid dermatitis, or at least get you into an eye-care program that does not cause you problems.

The use test on the previous page is a way you can test yourself for an eye product sensitivity.

Allergy testing of a more detailed kind can be done by dermatologists and allergists. Experience has shown, however, that this is a difficult and often impracticable approach, since there are so many product ingredients and often they are not available as individual chemicals for testing.

TREATING EYELID DERMATITIS

For a simple and not so severe problem you can successfully treat yourself. The treatment is the same no matter what the cause of your eyelid dermatitis. Those individuals who experience a more severe problem, or for whom simple home treatments are not effective within ten days, should definitely consult a dermatologist.

THE TREATMENT

Apply .5 percent hydrocortisone products. They are available over the counter—no prescription required.

Apply the hydrocortisone at least twice daily. Four times is better.

Apply the hydrocortisone very sparingly. Use so little that it does not get into the eyes and is not apparent on the skin (or no more than barely apparent).

Use the *ointment* form of hydrocortisone. The ointment form is of petrolatum (Vaseline) consistency and is *not creamy*. The cream forms are fine but may themselves contain ingredients that can irritate sensitive eyelid skin. Ask your pharmacist for help here if you need it.

The safety, for use on eyelids, of nonprescription-strength hydrocortisone products may be of concern to you. Though the information in the package cautions against using these products around the eyes, they really are quite safe for *limited use* there, if you are very careful. Limit use of the product to ten days. If you are not cleared up by then, consult your dermatologist.

Try not to get any cortisone products *in* your eyes. If you do, wash it out immediately. If irritation develops, see a doctor.

Do not use *any* "cortisone" products (prescription or over-the-counter) on the eyelids regularly over a prolonged period. Serious injury to the eyes can occur.

If seborrheic dermatitis is the cause of your eyelid problem, be sure you are working to control the seborrheic dermatitis (see chapter 15). Controlling seborrheic dermatitis of the scalp and elsewhere on the face is a big help in clearing up seborrheic dermatitis of the eyelids.

PIGMENTATION PROBLEMS

18

Areas of facial skin darker or lighter than the normal skin color are a real bother to those who have them. And they are a real bother to dermatologists, who know they are so difficult to treat satisfactorily. This section will discuss all the common facial skin pigmentation problems (and some of the less common ones) and help you approach a solution for them.

MELASMA, HYPERPIGMENTATION, CHLOASMA, MASK OF PREGNANCY

Melasma is a deposition of pigment—more pigment than normal—in blotches in various areas of the face. It most commonly affects the area above the upper lip, the forehead, and the cheeks. It can affect any part of the face, but those mentioned are the most frequent sites.

NOTE: Do not confuse melasma with the brown spot called lentigo or age spot. If in doubt, read about lentigo in chapter 22.

Causes of Melasma

Pregnancy is often the cause. And it is likely the hormone changes of pregnancy that produce the pigment change.

Birth-control pills are another frequent cause of melasma. Again, hormone changes are likely to be responsible. The newer "low-dose" pills do not seem to be as prone to cause melasma, but still may in highly susceptible individuals.

Skin injury may produce *postinflammatory hyperpigmentation*. The translation of that is simply "increased pigmentation where the skin has been inflamed or injured." It may be the result of a burn, dermabrasion or skin "sanding," or an abrasion from any other cause.

145

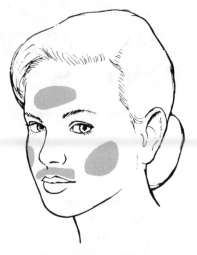

The pattern of melasma (pigmentation).

Especially in the very dark olive complexions and black skin, acne breakouts and even the use of too-strong acne medications may leave dark spots.

Some perfumes and colognes contain oils that, when applied to the skin and then exposed to the sun, may leave brown splotches. This happens in susceptible individuals only. This is much more common on the neck than the face, for perfume is more often applied to the neck.

Some women just have melasma for no known reason. Excess pigmentation may just be a product of that particular person's skin and sun exposure. And remember, you do not have to be a sunbather to get sun on your face. It is happening every day and every moment that you are exposed to outside light.

Things That Make Melasma Worse (Darker)

Pregnancy, birth-control pills, skin injury, of course, for they are the leading identifiable causes. But *sunlight* makes all cases of melasma, whatever the cause, much worse. Many women with melasma find it an easy problem to deal with in winter, when they are not getting much sun exposure—such a simple problem that it can be easily disguised with a little foundation make-up. But in summertime or any season when an individual gets more sun exposure, even if she is not trying to, the problem of melasma becomes a big one.

Any effort to treat melasma must be accompanied by a really strict effort to keep sun from hitting those dark areas. Even a little sun exposure may undo weeks of trying to bleach away the dark splotch.

Treating Melasma

There are two basic aspects to treating hyperpigmented areas of facial skin: pigment bleaching and absolute sun protection.

Pigment bleaching. All present bleaching agents, prescription or over-the-counter, contain *hydroquinone.* The products available only on a physician's prescription are more powerful and more effective.

NONPRESCRIPTION BLEACHES
Porcelana Medicated Fade Cream
Esoterica Medicated Fade Cream

PRESCRIPTION-ONLY BLEACHES
Melanex, an alcohol-based liquid
Solaquin Forte, a cream that also contains a sunblock
Eldoquin
Eldoquin Forte
Eldopaque

They all work. They all work *slowly.* Melanex is the current favorite of the authors. In an attempt to speed bleaching results, some derma-tologists are prescribing another medication (retinoic acid gel or cream) to be used along with the hydroquinone bleaching product. Whichever product you choose, use it diligently. *Apply it twice daily* to the pigmented areas. Use it just before makeup foundation is applied in the morning and before retiring at night.

Keep using it for a long time. It usually takes two months to notice a significant difference in the pigmentation. After the desired pig-ment-lightening effect has been achieved, it is well to continue a less frequent application schedule to those areas which give the most trouble. Certainly, start applications again at the first sign of pigment returning. However, the following should be noted:

1. Some individuals become sensitized (allergic) to any hydro-quinone bleaching product. It is wise to test for this before using it on the face. To do this, apply a little bit to a spot on the inner arm twice daily for a week. If it irritates the skin, do not use it on the face. Instead, consult your dermatologist.

Irritation on the face from using a bleaching product is likewise reason to discontinue its use and ask your dermatologist about it.

2. A few individuals can lose too much color with use of a bleaching agent. If skin areas are becoming white instead of your normal skin color, discontinue use and consult your dermatologist.

3. If you are under treatment for an acne problem, do not use hydroquinone bleaching products along with a benzoyl peroxide acne product. The combination of these two may produce an unsightly (temporary) brown stain on the skin—the last thing you want!

Sun protection. It is absolutely essential to protect yourself from sun exposure. *An hour of sun exposure can undo weeks of work with a bleaching product.* You cannot be successful in bleaching melasma unless you work very hard at sun protection. Here's how:

1. Apply a sunblock to the pigmented areas. Use a product with an SPF of 30 or higher. Use it after the bleaching agent is applied and before makeup is applied. *Never leave the house without it.*

2. Do wear foundation makeup. All makeup bases protect against the sun to some degree. Those with titanium dioxide seem to block sun, but are a bit heavier and more opaque. Those that contain sunscreens *may* be more effective. But read more about them in chapter 12. If you do not wear foundation, use your sunblock preparation several times daily.

3. Do not sunbathe the face, accidentally or on purpose. Just do not. Hats help and sunblocks help, but not enough. You just cannot do many sunny outdoor things—summer or winter—if you expect satisfactory results from a bleaching agent.

   Dermatologists would like to see the pharmaceutical industry develop a better bleaching agent, one that is more effective and faster. But with persistent use of today's bleaching agents and good sun protection, you can be helped—you just have to work hard at it.

WHITE AREAS OF FACIAL SKIN—HYPOPIGMENTATION

Pityriasis Alba

Translated, this means "scaling white areas." These usually appear only on the cheeks. They are most common in childhood but may persist into adulthood. They often appear scaly and whitish in the summer. They are generally an inch or more across and oval in shape. A frequent complaint is that these areas will not "tan" as well as the rest of the face.

Causes of pityriasis alba. Pityriasis alba just seems to be normal for some skin types. The individual affected usually has sensitive, easily dried out, and easily irritated skin. There is often a history of asthma or hayfever-type allergies in the individual or in family members.

Treating pityriasis alba. The approach most dermatologists take is a combination of lubrication and topical cortisone medication. Here is how you can do that:

1. Apply .5 percent hydrocortisone cream several times daily. Keep doing it until any sign of scale or irritation is gone—it usually requires no more than one week. This medication is available at your pharmacy, no prescription required.
2. Use moisturizers, any you like. After hydrocortisone cream has taken away the scale and irritation, moisturizers alone will likely keep it from returning. *Never* let the cheeks get dried out or chapped. This is important. Work especially hard at this during times of low humidity—during wintertime— and especially during winter outdoor activities.
3. The next step is a little sunshine to stimulate the return of the normal pigment. After all signs of scale and irritation are gone, sunshine *may* stimulate the return of pigment. The word "may" is used because in some individuals it is very slow.

Vitiligo

Vitiligo is a loss of pigment in areas all over the body, not just the face. It may affect any part of the face, but the skin around the eyes is the most common area.

Vitiligo affects the skin more or less *symmetrically*—that is, both eyes, both elbows, both knees, etc. The spots are smooth (no scale) and dead white. Vitiligo may (and usually does) become more extensive with time. The cause of vitiligo is simply not known. It seems to be hereditary in some cases.

Vitiligo is a difficult problem, though it can be treated with some success. The treatment is usually long and slow and must be carried out under the care of a dermatologist. If you think you have vitiligo, consult a dermatologist, who can better explain the nature of this problem and advise you of treatment options.

Camouflaging vitiligo. This condition can be minimized and even completely masked with makeup. For milder cases or for lighter complexions, a regular makeup foundation that gives a heavy coverage, such as Clinique's Continuous Coverage, Max Factor Pan-Stick, or Merle Norman Total Finish, among others, may do the trick for you. For more extensive cases, there are special camouflage cosmetics, such as Lydia O'Leary's Covermark, Dermablend's Dermablend Cover Cream, Max Factor's Erace, and Ar-Ex's Disappear, containing opaque masking agents—titanium dioxide and/or zinc oxide—that cover up skin discoloration. These products are waterproof and sunproof, but they are not perfect. It may be hard to find a perfect match for your complexion, for one thing. For another, these makeups tend to be very thick and may aggravate acne.

For best results, you should apply these makeups differently than you would a foundation. Dot them lightly on the affected areas and let it dry. Set the masker in place with translucent powder, then apply your usual foundation. For a "no-makeup" look, lightly brush loose powder over the camouflaged areas and the rest of your face.

In many cases, camouflage or coverup cosmetic treatment is the most practical approach.

Skin dyes are available, which can give coverage for several days. They must be applied carefully—several coats, maybe, until the correct shade is reached. Reapply when the color begins to wear away.

Nonprescription products, such as Vitadye and Dy O Derm, are available from your pharmacist.

FACIAL BLOOD VESSELS

19

They're often referred to as "broken veins," but they are not broken at all. These tiny, threadlike blood vessels are simply permanently dilated and very close to the surface, visible through the very thin stratum corneum. There are two types of dilated facial blood vessels.

SPIDER ANGIOMA (NEVUS ARANEUS, VASCULAR SPIDER)

This lesion is formed by a central vessel perpendicular to the skin surface and smaller vessels radiating from it. The central vessel is the body of the spider; the radiating vessels are the legs.

Vascular spiders may be congenital—showing up in infancy—or they may show up anywhere on the face at any time. They often show up during pregnancy.

PLAIN OLD DILATED BLOOD VESSELS

They are usually tiny, red, and threadlike, but may be larger and bluish. Favorite sites of development are around the nostrils, the cheekbone areas, and the nose itself. These plain old dilated veins are much more common in blonds and redheads than in those of darker skin tones. They are much more common in individuals of light skin tones who have had more than enough sun exposure. They are more common in individuals who flush and blush easily. They are more common in individuals whose parents had them.

151

What To Do About Dilated Facial Blood Vessels

They can be toned down or even completely camouflaged with makeup. In general, you'll need a coverup cream that matches your complexion, buy one that's opaque rather than sheer. Some suggestions: Clinique Continuous Coverage, Lydia O'Leary Covermark, Shading Cream, or Camouflage Crayon. For really red areas, dab on a green toner. Shiseido's Green Moisture Mist Compact Foundation tones down ruddiness. For other product suggestions, see chapter 12. Makeup is, of course, only a temporary measure.

A more permanent solution to both spider angiomas and plain old dilated veins is eradication by electric needle, or electrodessication. A fine, flexible needle is inserted into the vein. The electric current destroys the tiny vessel so no more blood can enter. That's how electrodessication gets the red out! By using this same principle, a finely aimed medical laser can also be used to treat dilated facial blood vessels.

20

PERIORAL DERMATITIS

This fancy-sounding name translates simply as "irritated skin around the mouth." No one knows why it occurs only around the mouth. It is somewhat baffling to doctors and may be *very* annoying to the individual who has it. For it is a skin problem of unknown cause, which may be *very* persistent, unsightly, and difficult to clear up.

The condition usually occurs in young adults (twenty- to thirty-year age group). It is sometimes seen in teenage years and also past thirty. The skins of the individuals who have it are usually of the sensitive type and also somewhat oily. It is often seen in individuals who have some acne tendency.

WHAT DOES IT LOOK LIKE?

It usually forms patches of red, bumpy, maybe scaly skin. It feels stingy and irritated.

Perioral dermatitis has ups and downs, gets worse and better, may fade away only to return. It lasts for a variable period—from months to years—until one day it just goes away and does not return.

TREATMENT

It is probably going to require a trip to the dermatologist to get this problem cleared up. Though there are some things an individual can do that may help, antibiotics of the tetracycline family (which require a doctor's prescription), taken by mouth, seem to be the most dependable method of controlling this problem. There are some

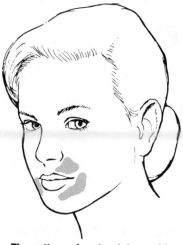

The pattern of perioral dermatitis.

topical agents (which require a doctor's prescription) that are useful, too.

SOME DO'S AND DON'TS

Don't use moisturizers or a makeup with a moisturizing base. Perioral dermatitis feels dry, but moisturizers seem to make it worse.

Don't use cortisone creams or ointments on this problem. The very mild .5 percent hydrocortisone products that can be bought without a prescription will not do any harm, but the powerful prescription ones will. These medications seem to help the problem but in the end make it much worse. If powerful cortisone medications have been used on this problem, they must be stopped. Stopping the use of these medications will probably result in worsening of the condition. This worsening simply must be lived through.

Don't rub these patches of dermatitis. Rubbing and fingering make the problem worse.

Do try a very mild acne medication, such as Komed, Komed Mild, or Rezamid, on the affected areas overnight and a tiny bit of .5 percent hydrocortisone lotion in the morning. Be patient (it takes at least a week to see results) and persistent with this medicating routine.

Do get some sun. Though sun may seem to make perioral dermatitis worse at first, it usually helps in the long run.

Do see a dermatologist. Perioral dermatitis usually needs professional help.

ROSACEA (ACNE ROSACEA) 21

Rosacea is an annoying skin problem that is not well understood by medical science. Rosacea causes redness, dilated blood vessels, and pimples and pustules on the nose and the entire central part of the face.

THE NATURE OF THE PROBLEM

Rosacea affects primarily individuals who are age fifty and beyond, but it can develop earlier than that. Both men and women are susceptible. It usually develops slowly, first on the nose, then spreading to the cheeks and forehead. It may affect the eyelid margins. The primary signs of rosacea are redness, pustules, and dilated blood vessesl.

Rosacea is a *chronic* problem, lasting nearly forever. It has its ups and downs. It may be (and usually is) a problem of only moderate severity. However, there are severe cases that, if left untreated, may advance to a cosmetic problem of major proportions. Rosacea is usually quite controllable if treated properly, but not curable (a cure means that, once treated, it stays away forever). It takes some effort and persistent medicating, but rosacea can usually be cleared up and kept that way.

The Rosacea Profile

Almost all cases of rosacea have the following characteristics in common:

Blushing and flushing facial skin
A history of acne

155

Fair complexion coloring
At least moderately oily skin

Women just after menopause or just after stopping female-hor-more (estrogen) therapy seem especially susceptible. Men and women who have significant or severe acne that persists into the thirty- to forty-year age bracket may also gradually develop rosacea as the acne fades.

THE CAUSE OF ROSACEA

The cause of rosacea is unknown. Many theories have been suggested. The most popular theory now is that repeated and continual flushing and blushing (dilation and contraction of facial blood vessels) is the cause. The blood vessels gradually lose their ability to contract; they stay dilated, so permanent redness occurs; and this is followed by the other signs of rosacea—pustules, pimples, and visibly dilated blood vessels.

The tendency to flushing and blushing is, like many other characteristics, inherited, so it may be said that the tendency to rosacea is inherited. A rapid drop in female-hormone levels (for example, after menopause or after stopping estrogen treatment) seems to trigger rosacea in many cases.

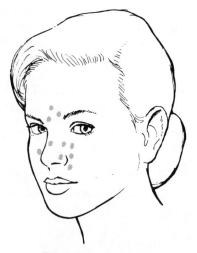

The pattern of rosacea.

Things That Aggravate Rosacea

The following factors may or may not play a role in *causing* rosacea, but they can surely make it worse and more difficult to control. All of the following factors tend to cause flushing of facial skin:

Alcoholic beverages
Heat—hot water, hot weather, hot foods, hot drinks
Spicy foods
Chocolate, tomatoes, citrus—anything that causes facial flushing
   in the individual

TREATING (CONTROLLING) ROSACEA

Remember that no treatment is going to really *cure* rosacea, though proper treatment can clear rosacea and keep it clear as long as the treatment is continued.

Effective treatment for rosacea is more than likely going to come from your dermatologist. There are some home medications and other help discussed below, but prescription drugs and expert care are almost always needed.

Tetracycline or another antibiotic taken by mouth is far and away the most effective treatment for rosacea. It should be taken at the recommended dosage until the problem is quiet. The dosage then may be reduced to the lowest required to keep the problem under control. One alternative is to stop the medication and start it again at the first sign of a flare-up. Most individuals learn how their rosacea problem responds to medications and what dosage schedule seems best for them.

There are some prescription topical medications—antibiotics and others—that when regularly applied to the skin are of value in treating rosacea. Your dermatologist will advise you about this.

Some Home Treatments for Rosacea

If your rosacea problem is not so severe and if you want to try treating yourself with available nonprescription medications, here is what to use and how to use it:

Sulfur acne medications can be very helpful. Try a mild one like Rezamid lotion or Komed lotion. Apply a thin film to the rosacea-prone areas overnight and keep doing it.

If you find that too drying, ask your pharmacist to mix for you *1 percent precipitated sulfur* in a cream base, such as Dermovan or Velvacol. Use it once or twice daily.

Miconazole nitrate 2 percent cream (Micatin cream, sold as an antifungal agent) is also helpful in some cases. This product will be better tolerated on the face if mixed half-and-half with a light moisturizing lotion, such as Nutraderm or Moisturel.

No matter what topical medication you are using, it is important that you understand the following points: Be consistent, regular, and persistent. Never miss a day of medication application. Apply the medication to the entire facial areas that are prone to rosacea outbreaks, not just to the lesions. Even when clear, continue medication applications, for *prevention* of those outbreaks is the goal. Read again the list of factors that aggravate rosacea and avoid them. Do the best you can.

An Important Note of Caution

Cortisone creams and ointments—those marvelous steroid preparations good for so many itchy rashes—are a really big no-no in rosacea. These products may seem to help at first, relieving the redness and clearing the pimples. But in the long run they make rosacea much worse and much more difficult to bring under control. Topical steroid preparations may even *cause* rosacea when used for too long in an attempt to clear some other facial rash. You may be one of those individuals who happen to have one of these creams in the medicine cabinet and decide to give it a try. Don't.

The cortisone creams you can buy without a doctor's prescription (.5 percent hydrocortisone) can be useful *on occasion* in helping take the redness out of a case of rosacea. But prolonged or regular use of any over-the-counter cortisone preparation is not recommended for rosacea. Remember *never* to use any prescription-strength cortisone preparations on rosacea.

COSMETICS AND SKIN CARE FOR ROSACEA

Cleansing. Use cool water (always) and a very gentle, lathering cleansing product. Examples are Dove bar, Aveeno bar, and Marcelle Gentle Cream Soap.

Covering the red of rosacea. Even if the rosacea outbreaks are quiet, the redness may remain. There are green moisturizers and makeup undercoats made specifically to camouflage red. The green color effectively masks the red of rosacea. Ask at your cosmetic counter, and see chapter 12 for some product suggestions.

Foundations. The lighter the better. Rosacea-prone skin does better if not heavily covered. Use an oil-free product if you can. Otherwise, select a *light* oil-containing one, and use it sparingly.

FACIAL GROWTHS AND SPOTS

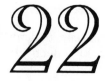

Make no mistake: You simply cannot learn to accurately diagnose facial growths and spots from this book. For any spot or growth not examined by a dermatologist or for any change in one that has been seen, consult a dermatologist. Taking chances with self-diagnosis in this area is very risky.

The following facial lesions are often asked about in the dermatologist's office.

Warts

Warts on the face are usually small, flat, and smooth. They tend to spread, giving rise to sometimes hundreds of small lesions on the face. They may not look like regular warts, because often they do not have the typical rough elevated surface.

They are difficult to cure, even for your dermatologist. Various treatments are available from your doctor. Often, more than one must be tried for successful removal.

All warts are caused by a virus. If you have facial warts, you may have contaminated your cosmetic and skin-care products with the virus by using your fingers for application. It is a good idea to get new products and avoid contaminating them by using a spoon to dip out what you need for that application. Warts can be contagious. Close face-to-face contact may cause warts on the face of another person. Be careful.

Molluscum Contagiosum

This is another viral problem of facial skin. The lesions of molluscum contagiosum (MC) are small, round, and pearly, and have a tiny dimple on the top.

Like warts, MC may be contagious, may spread around the face, and may contaminate makeup containers. And as with warts, your dermatologist has effective treatment methods.

Age Spots, Lentigo, Liver Spots

These brown spots appear on some faces as a result of time and sun exposure. They are not elevated above the skin surface and thus have no "feel." They are benign spots but may on rare occasions take a malignant turn. Be alert for darker areas developing in these lesions and consult a dermatologist immediately if that happens. These spots can be lightened using bleaching agents, but they can be removed much faster by a dermatologist.

Seborrheic Keratosis, Moles

These lesions can appear anywhere on the face, but the hairline is the favorite spot. They are elevated from the skin surface, have a slightly rough texture, and at times may be crumbly. They are tan, brown, gray, or black. They may be very small or quite large. They appear more often with advancing age, but may occur in younger individuals, too.

They are benign lesions of unknown causation. They are surface lesions, appearing almost as though they were "stuck on." Because of their superficial nature, they are quite easily removed. Ask your dermatologist.

Actinic Keratosis, Solar Keratosis, Senile Keratosis

"Actinic" and "solar" mean "from sunlight"; "senile" means "from old age." These lesions are definitely caused by sun exposure. They may definitely appear on individuals before old age. Individuals with fair skin who get too much sun are definitely more susceptible to developing actinic keratosis than are those of darker complexion or those who protect themselves from sun exposure.

Actinic keratoses are red with rough or spiny-feeling scales on them. They are usually about half an inch in diameter, but may be larger or smaller. They are *premalignant* lesions and will eventually develop into skin cancers, so they should be removed. Since they are superficial, they are easily removed. Individuals who are prone to the development of these lesions should visit a dermatologist at least yearly.

Moles, Nevi

These are the usual brown moles that start in childhood or teenage years and gradually enlarge. They have smooth surfaces, may or may not have hairs growing from them, and may or may not be elevated above the skin surface.

Nevi ("nevus" is the singular) may be easily removed if they are a cosmetic bother. Be alert to any change in a mole. Always have a dermatologist examine any mole that has changed in any way. Do this as soon as you notice a change; do not delay. Though it is rare, moles may turn cancerous; and, when they do, they develop into a very serious melanoma, which is the most dangerous type of skin cancer. You should also see a physician immediately if you have a mole larger than a quarter inch in diameter, one of irregular shape, one of a very dark color, or one that is more than one color.

Sebaceous Hyperplasia

"Sebaceous" means "oil gland"; "hyperplasia" means "overgrowth." So these lesions are caused by an overgrowth of oil glands. This overgrowth forms small yellowish bumps on the face. The forehead is the favorite spot for them. They are always seen in individuals with very oily skin. Other than that, their cause is unknown. They may be easily removed or at least made less noticeable by simple procedures performed by your dermatologist.

Cherry Angiomas, Senile Angiomas

These are tiny cherry red spots, usually smooth and slightly elevated from the skin's surface. They are caused by an overgrowth of tiny blood vessels. They are benign.

Basal Cell Carcinoma

This is the most common skin cancer, far and away more common than any other type. It appears as a small pearly or waxy bump, then enlarges and develops a sunken area in its center. The center may ulcerate and bleed. Close examination usually reveals tiny blood vessels coursing over the surface of a basal cell carcinoma.

This lesion only very rarely metastasizes, or spreads through the body, but it is locally destructive. Basal cell carcinoma is almost always easily curable with a minor surgical procedure.

Squamous Cell Carcinoma

This is the kind of skin cancer that develops from actinic keratosis. This lesion is usually hard and has a "horny" feeling. It may develop anywhere on the face—even the lip. Squamous cell carcinoma is more serious than basal cell carcinoma, especially when it is on the lip. These lesions are usually completely curable by simple surgical treatment, but they should be treated early to prevent spread.

These are the most common facial growths and spots. There are many other kinds that only dermatologists know about. The advice given at the beginning of this chapter is repeated here: For any new spot or growth or for any change in an old one, consult a dermatologist for an expert opinion.

FACIAL HAIR 23

Male hormone levels—and perhaps the relative amounts of male and female hormones—are important factors in facial hair growth. Males have beards due to their high levels of male hormones. But those with heavy beards do not necessarily have higher male hormone levels than those with lighter beards. Why? Because heredity and racial origin play a very prominent role in determining the heaviness of facial hair. Hormonally normal men may have heavy beards or very sparse ones, depending on the genetic traits of their parents.

Females have facial hair, and here, too, the amount and kinds of facial hair are determined by hormone levels, heredity, and racial origin. Females may have more facial hair than desired and be (and usually are) perfectly normal hormonally.

The question is how to tell when your facial hair problem is "normal" and needs to be dealt with using cosmetic measures, and when it is "abnormal" and needs medical attention because it is due to a hormone problem.

NORMAL OR ABNORMAL?

Downy Facial Hair

Downy facial hair is usually normal, even if it is heavier than you like. We see this type of hair most commonly on the cheeks, especially in the "sideburn" areas, and above the upper lip.

The amount of downy facial hair one has is almost always genetically determined and not caused by hormone imbalances. In other words, downy facial hair, even if it is more than you want, is probably just normal for you. Deal with the downy hair problem as suggested below.

164

The color of downy facial hair has a great deal to do with its visibility and therefore whether it is a cosmetic problem. The color parallels the color of head hair and other body hair, and therefore has no significance as to whether it is normal or abnormal for you. Sometimes simple bleaching is adequate cosmetic treatment here. See suggestions later.

Excessive amounts of downy facial hair *can* be a sign of hormonal abnormality. If you have a true excess, and really can't find the problem in your family tree, have it checked out by a dermatologist, gynecologist, or endocrinologist. This is especially important if you have any other signs of hormone problems, such as acne, infertility, or irregularity or absence of menstrual periods.

Wiry or Whiskerlike Facial Hair

Wiry or whiskerlike facial hair is usually seen on the chin area. It is often associated with a hormonal change (especially after menopause) or a real hormone abnormality (an excessive production of male hormones). Whisker-like hair is also influenced by heredity. For example, if your mother or grandmother developed significant chin hair after menopause, you may also.

The development of wiry hairs, especially on the chin after menopause, is usually considered normal. This problem can be helped by the suggestions below. But if excessive whiskerlike facial hair develops, even after menopause, it should be investigated by a dermatologist, gynecologist, or endocrinologist.

Wiry facial hair developing before menopause, especially in the twenty- to forty-year old group, is a definite signal to have a medical evaluation of the problem. Absence or irregularity of menstrual periods, infertility, the development of facial or body acne, and the development of excessive body hair are also symptoms of hormone problems.

If you have excess hair and want to know how to get rid of it, here are some hair-removal options:

MECHANICAL METHODS

Shaving

Despite the decidedly unfeminine connotation of shaving your face, this method is quick, easy, and inexpensive. The downside: Hair grows back within a few days. That means you have to keep it up once you've started—and skin can get irritated. To get a smooth, close shave:

• *Use the proper tool.* For limited areas on the face, you'll get the most cosmetic results with a hand razor, not an electric one. It gives a smoother, more precise result.

• *Prep your face.* The area to be shaved should be moistened (see below) and covered with a lathering soap or shaving cream—this protects the skin from unsightly nicks.

• *Time your shave properly.* Shave before you bathe or shower. Prolonged soaking plumps up skin and you won't be able to shave as closely. Try not to shave before swimming or sunning, which can irritate vulnerable skin.

• *Use the best shaving technique.* Shave with a light hand (pressure can scrape and irritate skin), using long upward strokes *against* the direction of hair growth.

• *Be sure to change razors* or razor blades regularly. Dulled edges mean more strokes, and scraping over the area again and again can leave it red and rashy.

• *Take care of your razor.* After each use, rinse it thoroughly in hot water and shake off the water. Don't wipe the blade, as this dulls it.

• *Care for your skin after shaving* with a mild lotion—one that doesn't contain alcohol. Shaving scrapes away some of the protection stratum corneum, and alcohol can sting this sensitive skin.

ONCE AND FOR ALL: DEBUNKING THE MYTH THAT SHAVING MAKES HAIR GROW BACK COARSER, THICKER, DARKER

It just doesn't, for this simple reason: The normal hair shaft is widest at the middle and tapers toward the end. When you shave, you're cutting the hairs at their widest point, not at their narrower end. So when hair starts regrowing, it *looks* coarser, thicker, perhaps darker. Shaving does not permanently change the character of your hair.

Waxing

Waxing consists of applying a thin layer of heated, melted wax to the skin and allowing it to cool and solidify, embedding the hairs. There is also a cold wax method (called "zipping") in which sticky wax, then a cloth strip are pressed over the area to be bared. The wax is then removed by pulling in the direction of hair growth. Waxing can be done professionally as well as at home.

This method is typically used for the upper and lower lip, the sides of the cheeks (in the sideburn area), and on the chin. Results last for three to six weeks, but hair must grow out until it is long enough for the wax to grab on to it again. That means that excess hair will be visible for a short time before waxing can be redone. To cope with hair in this in-between phase, you may try bleaching. (See "Chemical Methods," on page 168)

Waxing removes hair by the roots, but the hair-producing bulb remains intact, so another hair can and does sprout. Over time, the bulbs may become damaged, so that long-term waxing may cause some thinning of the regrowing hair. Waxing can be painful (especially on the upper lip, which is full of nerve endings) and can cause ingrown hairs.

For professional results at home:

• *Dust the area* to be waxed with baby powder before applying wax. This protects the skin.

• *Afterward,* smoothe on a gentle moisturizer to calm skin.

• *For hot wax products,* test the temperature by dabbing a bit on the inner forearm. Too-hot wax can cause serious burns.

Some effective drugstore products: Zip Depilatory Wax, Better Off Natural Wax Hair Remover and Dorothy Gray Wax (hot waxes), and Cosmagique's Hair Off and Sally Hansen's Hair Removal System (cold wax strips).

Tweezing

This is a very effective method for removing stray wiry hairs that may crop up on the sides of cheeks or the chin or grow from moles. This method is a good choice if you have a relatively small number of hairs. If you're patient, tweezing can clear small well-defined areas of fine, downy hairs as well (a patch of hairs on the chin or a clearly visible area of the cheek, for instance). It yields the same weeks-long smoothness as waxing. Swabbing the area to be tweezed with an alcohol-containing astringent or witch hazel, and tweezing in the direction of hair growth can reduce any discomfort.

Tweezing mole hairs does not cause cancer or cause moles to turn malignant, but a mole may become irritated from the traction pressure. If this is the case, try clipping hairs off at the surface until the irritation clears. Another choice is having your physician simply remove the mole.

CHEMICAL METHODS

Bleaching

Bleaching works best on fine but dark hair that occurs on the sides of cheeks and the upper lip. It's simple, inexpensive, and painless; but it's not for everyone. Those with lighter complexions get the most cosmetic results from bleaching—the less of a contrast between skin and bleached hairs, the more natural the result.

Commercial preparations contain hydrogen peroxide and alkali (usually ammonia) to augment the bleaching powers of the hydrogen peroxide. Jolen Cream Bleach, Sally Hansen Extra Strength Creme Bleach, and Nudit Cream Bleach for the Face are fine to use.

For best bleaching results:

• *Patch-test* with a small amount on the inner arm. Leave it on for thirty minutes. If no redness or other irritation develops, go ahead and bleach the desired area.

• *Apply moisturizer* after bleaching to keep skin irritation at a minimum. For very sensitive skin, nonprescription hydrocortisone creams are more effective anti-irritants.

• *To go still lighter,* wait two days and bleach again. Don't leave bleach on for longer than the recommended time. You won't lighten hair any more and may irritate the skin. Rebleaching is really important if the first application turns your dark facial hair red instead of the desired colorless hue.

Depilatories

These let you lotion, cream, spray, or foam away unwanted hair. These products chemically dissolve hair at the skin surface and, perhaps, just below the skin line. Results last about as long as shaving (maybe a day longer). The chemicals (usually sulfides or thioglycol-lates break down the sulfur bonds in hair proteins, so hair can be wiped away. Sulfide-containing products have a distinct "rotten egg" odor, but are stronger and more effective, and more likely to cause skin irritation than thioglycollate-containing products. Sulfide ones usually contain some scent (lemon, cocoa butter) to mask the sulfide odor, but such scents may be irritating in and of themselves. Thioglycollate ones have to be left on longer but aren't as irritating or odorous.

For best results:

• *Patch-test* any product before using it. Apply on the inner forearm for the time recommended in the directions, rinse, and check the spot a day later. A little irritation here may be tolerable, but a strong reaction to this test means stay away from this method of hair removal.

• *Use a timer.* The most common flub, when it comes to using a depilatory, is leaving it on too long. The chemicals can be highly irritating to skin. Read the directions, and time your application precisely. The rash that can result form overdoing a depilatory is more noticeable than the hair you're trying to get rid of.

• *Follow up* with something to soothe skin. A moisturizer may be enough, but a nonprescription hydrocortisone cream is a much more effective soothing choice. Use .5 percent hydrocortisone cream twice daily before the depilatory and twice daily for two days after treatment.

• *Use a facial depilatory.* Those for body hair are much more potent and potentially more irritating to facial skin. Ones to try: Sally Hansen Roll-on Hair Remover (with vitamin E), Sally Hansen Facial Hair Cream Remover, Nudit Cream Hair Remover, One Touch Roll On Depilatory (in regular and sensitive-skin formulas), Neet Cream Hair Remover, Better Off Facial Hair Remover Cream, and Ardell SurgiCream Cream Depilatory.

ELECTROLYSIS

Electrolysis offers permanent hair removal. Treatment consists of inserting a fine needle into a hair follicle and destroying the hair bulb with a momentary (one twentieth of a second) burst of electricity. What does it feel like? It depends on you and your threshold of pain, but it has been described variously as a twinge, a prickle, or a zap. The process is time-consuming (hairs must be treated one by one), and it can only remove those hairs in the active growing phase—only about half of the hairs you see. (The rest are in dormant or transitional phases.) The area must be touched up monthly to treat all hairs in their growth phases. That translates as six to eight months' worth of treatment. At around fifty dollars per session, electrolysis is expensive up-front, but can save you hours and expense over the long term. (Think of it, never having to buy a depilatory, bleach, or razor again!)

There are also some valid health concerns associated with electrolysis—in the hands of an unskilled operator, electrolysis can result in permanent scarring or pigmentation changes. And though no cases have been reported, it is theoretically possible to transfer hepatitis, herpes, or the AIDS virus via an unsterilized needle. Don't hesitate to ask about sterilization practices before you start electrolysis. Many clients buy their own needle probes for their exclusive use.

How to choose an electrologist? Get a recommendation from a dermatologist or endocrinologist; insist on an electrologist with a certificate from a recognized electrology training institution.

As for the big electrolysis turnoff—pain, there are some tips to reduce the discomfort level:

- *Take two aspirins* (or ibuprofen, the aspirin substitute) twenty to thirty minutes prior to your appointment, to reduce minor pain.
- *Don't schedule appointments before or just after your period* (three or four days either way). Body tissue retains more fluid than usual around this time, and this can increase discomfort.
- *Schedule electrolysis early in the day.* As the day goes on, body tissues accumulate fluids.
- *Arrive on time* for your appointment—rushing to the appointment, arriving nervous and anxious, can make you tense and more sensitive to electrolysis.
- *Ask the operator to periodically swab on a mild topical antiseptic* to reduce discomfort.
- *Ask the operator to take a break* if you feel the discomfort is too much. You're in control; don't feel you have to submit.
- After treatment, you'll notice tiny flea-bite type welts in the treatment area—these are the skin's reaction to the current. They clear up in about thirty minutes. If the upper lip is being treated, hot compresses applied three times daily for two to three days after a treatment can prevent whiteheads and irritation that might develop in this sensitive area. An application of nonprescription hydrocortisone cream before and just after treatment, and twice daily for the next two days, can really reduce irritation and redness. To guard against infection, a very think film of antibiotic ointment (Polysporin, Neosporin, Mycitracin) can be used along with the hydrocortisone cream.

IN CONCLUSION

Just how face-smart are you? Having read every—or even one—chapter in this book has made you that much smarter about your skin: the care, the techniques, the routines, the products that it needs to look great, now and later on.

But learning doesn't stop here. This book is just a start. Ongoing research, both in skin-specific fields as well as general ones, will continue to turn up new facts about this largest organ of the human body. Cosmetics companies are constantly refining formulas to make better, more effective products. If no cosmetic is completely breakout-proof in 1988, you can bet there will be some strong contenders in the coming years. Part of the reason for the continued growth in knowledge is due to an informed consumer—that's you—demanding safe, effective products and truth in advertising. So it's to your advantage to be as face-smart as you can be.

This book contains the basics pertaining to the function and the maintenance of skin, which you can refer to again and again. The *skin's structure* (chapter 2) is no mystery anymore, and that knowledge has thrown new light on some old tenents. You now know that the tissue-paper-thin top layer of skin is such an effective barrier that cosmetic and skin-care products cannot penetrate it. You know that surface conditions such as *wrinkles* (chapter 3) and *large pores* (chapter 4) result from changes in the deeper layers of skin—wrinkles from damage and weakness in the deepest layer of skin, and large pores from the underlying oil glands. You know the difference between *dry skin* (chapter 5) and *oily skin* (chapter 6), that dry isn't the opposite of oily and that oily skin can often be confused with dry skin. You also know where your skin falls in the dry-to-oily spectrum.

Understanding your skin leads to informed skin care—which products to use and how to use them. You can now decode *advertising claims* (chapter 7) to purchase the particular *sun-protection products* (chapter 8), *cleansing products* (chapter 9), *treatment products and services* (chapter 10), *moisturizers* (chapter 11), *foundations, blush-*

ers, and powders (chapter 12) and *anti-aging products* (chapter 13) that are right for your skin and your budget.

Over and above cosmetic skin care, there's medical skin care. You now have a handle on some of the problems that can occur: *acne* (chapter 14), *seborrheic dermatitis* (chapter 15), *cosmetic reactions* (chapter 16), *eyelid dermatitis* (chapter 17), *pigmentation problems* (chapter 18), *facial blood vessels* (chapter 19), *perioral dermatitis* (chapter 20), *rosacea* (chapter 21), *facial growths and spots* (chapter 22), and *facial hair* (chapter 23). You can make an informed decision as to when it's appropriate to treat yourself with over-the-counter medications and when it's time to consult a dermatologist; taking advantage of his or her training, expertise, and knowledge of prescription medications.

Congratulations! You are now a *Smart Face*.

APPENDIX
Consumer Product Information

Sunscreens

Product	Price ($–$$$)	Ingredients of Note	Skin Type	Comments
Sun Seekers Avon Ultra Sunsafe Sunblocking Lotion	$$	*	normal	PABA-free, water resistant
Biotherm Oil Free Sun Protector	$$$	*, padimate-O, oxybenzone	oily	light, nongreasy
Chanel Sun Shelter Cream Haute Protection	$$$	*, aloe, padimate-O, oxybenzone	sensitive	not greasy
Clarins Total Sunscreen	$$	*, octyl methoxycinnamate, oxybenzone, mineral oil	normal-sensitive	PABA-free, SPF 18
Coppertone Waterbabies Sunblock Lotion	$	*, methoxycinnamate, oxybenzone, salicylates, homosalate	sensitive, delicate	PABA-free, nonsting formula, nongreasy, waterproof
Coppertone Waterbabies Sun Cream	$	*, methoxycinnamate, oxybenzone, salicylates, homosalate	sensitive, delicate	SPF 25, PABA-free
Neutrogena Sunscreen	$$	*, ethylhexyl p-methoxycinnamate, oxybenzone	sensitive or dry	contains no alcohol
PreSun 29 Sensitive Skin Sunscreen	$$	*, methoxycinnamate, oxybenzone, octyl salicylate	sensitive, dry	waterproof

Product	Price	Active ingredient(s)	Skin type	Notes
Piz Buin Exclusiv Extrem (Greiter)	$$	*, octylmethoxycinnamate, benzophenone	sensitive, dry	waterproof, SPF 15
Solbar Lotion (Person & Covey)	$$	*, octyl dimethyl PABA, oxybenzone	sensitive, normal	comes in PABA-free formula, SPF 15
TiScreen Lotion (T/I Pharmaceuticals)	$$	*, methoxycinnamate, oxybenzone	dry, normal	PABA-free, SPF 15
Total Eclipse PABA-free Sunblock Lotion	$	*, methoxycinnamate, oxybenzone, salicylate	dry	creamy, not sticky
Nivea Moisturizing SunBlock Lotion (Beiersdorf)	$$	*, octyl methoxycinnamate, PABA esters	dry to normal	SPF 15 and SPF 25
Presun Facial Sunscreen (Westwood)	$$	*, octyl dimethyl PABA, oxybenzone	dry to normal	SPF 15, fragrance free
Sebastian Ultrablock	$$	*, oxybenzone	dry, normal	SPF 29
Estée Lauder Super Sun Block	$$$	*, octyl dimethyl PABA	normal-dry	SPF 20, moisturizing, long-lasting
Clinique Face Zone SunBlock	$$$	*, oxybenzone	normal-dry	SPF 15, may be OK for slightly oily faces
Elizabeth Arden Super Block	$$	*, PABA esters	normal	SPF 34

*In general, sunscreens contain an active ingredient (PABA), emollient (lanolin, isopropyl myristate, petrolatum), and preservatives (quaternium 15, propylparabens, citric acid).

Product	Price ($–$$$)	Ingredients of Note	Skin Type	Comments
Sea & Ski Block Out Sunblock Cream Lotion (Carter)	$	*, octyl dimethyl PABA, methoxycinnamate, salicylate	oily	doesn't exacerbate acne, SPF 30
PreSun 15 Lotion	$$	*, octyl dimethyl PABA, oxybenzone, SD alcohol 40	oily	long-lasting, cooling
Clinique Oil-Free Sun Block SPF 15	$$$	*, padimate-O	oily	won't stain clothing
Elizabeth Arden Sun Science Oil Free Ultra Block	$$$	*, padimate-O, oxybenzone	oily	SPF 15
Super Shade 15 (and 25) (Schering-Plough)	$	*, methoxycinnamate, salicylate, padimate-O, oxybenzone	normal	protects against UVA & B
Elizabeth Arden Superblock Cream 34	$$$	*, PABA esters	normal, mature	nongreasy
Sunblock Cream Sunblock Lotion Sunblock Stick (Johnson & Johnson)	$ $ $	*, octyl dimethyl PABA, oxybenzone (all)	dry oily dry skin areas (under eyes, ears)	SPF 24 SPF 20 SPF 20 all are basic and effective
Chanel Protection Extreme Sun Shelter Face Block	$$$	*, methoxycinnamate	dry or normal	solid concentrate with mirror compact handy for reapplication

176

Product	Price	Ingredients	Skin Type	Notes
Avon Sun Seekers Sunblocking Stick	$	*, padimate-O	dry, normal	long-lasting
Total Eclipse Lip and Face Sunscreen Protectant	$	*, PABA esters	all	long-lasting stick
PreSun 15 Sunscreen Stick	$$	*, PABA esters	all	good for oily skin, nonstaining
Bonnie Bell Weatherproofer	$	*, PABA esters	all	comes on a string to keep it handy
Le Zinc	$	*, zinc oxide, homosalate	all	opaque coverage in brights—yellow, blue, orange, pink
Coppertone Zinka Ztick (Schering-Plough)	$	*, zinc oxide	all	zinc oxide in colors
Clinique Continuous Coverage	$$$	no chemical sunscreens; talc, kaolin, mica	sensitive, normal	opaque cream, six shades
Estée Lauder Total Sunblock Cream	$$$	no chemical sunscreens	sensitive, normal	opaque cream, SPF 23

*In general, sunscreens contain an active ingredient (PABA), emollient (lanolin, isopropyl myristate, petrolatum), and preservatives (quaternium 15, propylparabens, citric acid).

Cleansers

Product	Price ($–$$$)	Ingredients of Note	Skin Type	Comments
Ponds Essential Cleansing Lotion	$	*, mineral oil	dry, mature	for other skin types, follow with lathering cleanser
Dorothy Gray Magic Moisturing Cleansing Cream	$	*, mineral oil, ozerkenite	dry, normal	effectively removes mascara as well as other makeup; thin consistency
Jergens All Purpose Face Cream	$	*, mineral oil	dry, normal	less greasy than most
Orlane Ligne Active Lait Demaquillant	$$$	*, mineral oil, stearic acid	normal, oily, not acne-prone	thick but not greasy
Germain Monteil Super Moist Cleansing Cream	$$	*, mineral oil, sorbitol stearate	dry, normal	can irritate sensitive eyes; not for contacts wearers
Lancôme Galatee Milky Creme Cleanser	$$$	*, mineral oil, isopropyl myristate	dry, normal	not for acne-prone skin; squeeze bottle, thin lotion
Doak Pharmaceutical Formula 405 Facial Cleansing Cream	$	*, DEA lauryl sulfate, fragrance	all except sensitive	polyurethane mitt may be too harsh for sensitive or very dry skin
Cetaphil Lotion	$	*, cetyl alcohol	dry-normal	light formula, good cleansing action

Product	Price	Ingredients	Skin Type	Comments
Almay Oil Control Facial Cleanser for Oily Skin	$	*, ammonium lauryl sulfate	oily	use in addition to or instead of soap and water for exceptionally oily skin
Aquanil Lotion	$	*	dry	gentle formula, good basic product
Lancôme Douceur Demaquillante Nutrix	$$	*, mineral oil, isopropyl palmitate	dry	may be too emollient for some
Clinique Extremely Gentle Cleansing Cream	$$	*, mineral oil, petrolatum, sterile alcohol, lanolin alcohol	normal	tissue or rinse off
Prescriptives Essential Cleansing Gel	$	*, sodium lauryth sulfate, cocoamidopropyl betaine	normal, oily	oil-free formula, gentle cleansing, fragrance-free
Contrôle de Lancôme Priming Cleanser for Oily Skin	$$$	*, witch hazel extract, diethylene glycol	oily	removes makeup well, including mascara; leaves skin clean, not greasy

*In general, a cleanser contains water, waxes, oils, and fats.

179

Lathering Cleansers

Product	Price ($–$$$)	Ingredients of Note	Skin Type	Comments
Ivory soap	$	•	normal, oily	may be too harsh for sensitive skin
Basis (Beiersdorf)	$	• (superfatted)	dry, normal	superfatted soap; also available in transparent glycerin form. May be too drying for very dry skin
Oilatum (Steifel)	$	•, sodium tallowate, peanut oil, lecithin	dry, normal	polyunsaturated vegetable oils leave skin soft
Eucerin Cleansing Bar (Beiersdorf)	$	•, triple pressed stearic acids, hydrogenated tallow fatty acids, "Eucerite"	dry, sensitive	good moisturizing properties, "Eucerite" is a combination of ingredients that mimic skin's natural oils
Neutrogena	$	•, glycerin	all	specific formulas for all skin types; nonirritating and effective, but dissolves quickly
Purpose (Johnson & Johnson)	$	•, glycerin, sodium salts of fatty acids	all	very gentle

Product	Price	Ingredients	Skin Type	Notes
Pears Transparent Soap	$	*, glycerin, cedar, thyme	normal, oily, dry	not too drying for dry or sensitive skin, also in liquid form
Neutrogena Liquid Facial Cleansing Formula	$	*, glycerin	normal	easily rinsed, same soap base as bar formulation
pHresh 3.5	$	*, cocamidopropyl betaine, lactic acid	normal to dry	nondrying soapless cleanser
Aveeno Bar	$	*, colloidal oatmeal, sulfur, salicylic acid	oily	good thorough cleanser, some exfoliative action
Erno Lazlo Hydraphel Cleansing Treatment	$$$	*	dry, delicate	lifts impurities without irritation
Jergens Clear Complexion Bar	$	*, glycerin, alcohol, lanolin	oily, acne-prone	effective cleanser; needs extra-thorough rinsing to remove completely
Clinique Facial Soap	$$	*, (superfatted)	extra strength–oily; mild–normal	thick lather; degreases skin well, may be too drying for dry skin
Lowila Cake (Westwood)	$	*, sodium lauryl sulfoacetate, boric acid, urea	sensitive	rich lather

*In general, a lathering cleanser contains water, waxes, oils, and fats.

Product	Price ($–$$$)	Ingredients of Note	Skin Type	Comments
Dove (Lever Bros.)	$	*, stearic acid, sodium tallowate, coconut oil	normal, dry	"one quarter cleansing cream"; leaves skin supple; rinse thoroughly
Bonnie Bell Ten-O-Six Cleansing Bar	$	*, resorcinol, allantoin	normal, oily	resorcinol may cause pigmentation problems in black or dark skin
Esteem Thorough Cleansing Bar	$	*, sodium lauryl sulfate, cornstarch	all	non-alkaline, gentle cleaner

Astringents

Product	Price ($–$$$)	Ingredients of Note	Skin Type	Comments
Clairol Sea Breeze Antiseptic	$	†, SD alcohol 40, camphor, peppermint, eucalyptus and clove oils	normal, oily	reduces oiliness
Clairol Sea Breeze Antiseptic for Sensitive Skin	$	†, benzethonium chloride, glycerin, benzoic acid	sensitive	non-irritating, non-drying formula
Dickinson's Witch Hazel	$	†, witch hazel, alcohol	normal, oily	strong odor, controls oiliness; very inexpensive
Almay Counter Balance Pore Lotion	$$	†, SD alcohol 40, polysorbate 80	oily, very oily	long-lasting reduction of oily feeling, shiny look

Product	Price	Ingredients	Skin Type	Notes
Almay Moisture Balance Toner	$	†, SD alcohol 40	normal	light formula
Almay Moisture Renewal Toner	$	†, SD alcohol 40	dry	non-irritating
Almay Oil Control Toner	$	†, SD alcohol 40, acetone	oily	good oil-stopper
Allercreme Astringent for Oily Skin	$	†, SD alcohol 40, acetone	oily	fragrance-free
Allercreme Skin Freshner	$	†, SD alcohol 40, propylene glycol, citric acid	normal	mild, not drying
Bonnie Bell Ten-O-Six Lotion	$	†, isopropyl alcohol, resorcinol, allantoin	normal, oily, acne-prone	can be diluted to meet your needs; resorcinol can cause pigmentation problems in black and dark skin
Lancôme Tonique Douceur	$$	†, rose water, glycerin, benzoic acid, castor oil	dry, sensitive, normal	alcohol-free, removes makeup, cleansing cream; leaves skin fresh and soft
Estée Lauder Mild Action Protection Tonic	$$	†, SD alcohol 40, allantoin	normal	not harsh, also in oily and dry skin formulas
Discipline Skin Care The Solution	$$	†, witch hazel	oily	mild astringent action

*In general, a lathering cleanser contains water, waxes, oils, and fats.
†In general, astringents contain water, alcohol, sometimes a mineral salt (aluminum/zinc) to blot oil, fragrance, cooling agent (camphor/menthol, mint, eucalyptus).

Product	Price ($–$$$)	Ingredients of Note	Skin Type	Comments
Clinique Clarifying Lotion	$$	•, SD alcohol 40, witch hazel, acetone	normal, oily, dry	formulas number 1, 2, 3; effective; come in glass bottles—not for butter fingers!; 3 is very good for the acne-prone

Scrubbers

Product	Price ($–$$$)	Ingredients of Note	Skin Type	Comments
Flori Roberts Derma Pure Facial	$$$	†, peanuts, honey	all	formulated for black skin; good basic product
Brasivol Lathering Scrub Cleanser	$	†, sodium lauryl sulfate, aluminum oxide particles	oily, acne-prone	available in fine, medium, and rough; very potent; label recommends not using other soaps/cleansers
Dorothy Gray Cleansing Grains	$	†, sodium tallowate, titanium dioxide, pumice	normal, oily	dry powder to be mixed with water, rinses away easily, less abrasive than others
Clairol Sea Breeze Facial Scrub	$	†, polyethylene, glycerine, camphor	normal, oily	oil-free, good for oily skins; whipped formulation
Revlon Moon Drops Sluffing Masque	$$	†, almond meal, walnut shell, mineral oil, petrolatum	oily	very abrasive, use carefully

Product	Price	Ingredients	Skin Type	Comments
Coty Sweet Earth "Suds"	$	†, myristic acid, pumice	sensitive, oily	very gentle; may not exfoliate enough for very oily skins
Biotherm Gentle Facial Scrub	$$$	†, butylene glycol	oily	mild action
Clinique 7th-Day Scrub Cream	$$$	†, mineral oil, beeswax, ozerkenite	sensitive, mature	gentle, cream-based formula
Clinique Exfoliating Scrub	$$$	†, cocoamphocarboxyglycinate, polyethylene	oily	water soluable; good for oily skin troubled by creamy formulations
Estée Lauder Gentle Action Skin Polisher	$$	†, mineral oil	normal, dry	grainy yet delicate
Adrien Arpel Honey & Almond Scrub	$$$	†, glycerine, honey, almond meal	normal, mildly oily	pleasant scent, leaves skin soft
Esteem Gentle Skin Sweeper	$$$	†, polyethylene	normal	gentle formula, creamy feel
Prescriptives Skin Refiner	$$$	†, mineral oil	normal	delicate, non-irritating yet effective; gel form for oily skin
Lancôme Bienfait Demaquillant	$$$	†, kaolin	mature, normal, slightly oily	clay base, masklike cleansing wash

*In general, astringents contain water, alcohol, sometimes a mineral salt (aluminum/zinc) to blot oil, fragrance, cooling agent (camphor/menthol, mint, eucalyptus).
†In general, scrubbers consist of an abrasive material (pumice, almond meal, apricot) in a base of lotion, cream, or soap.

185

Masks

Product	Price ($–$$$)	Ingredients of Note	Skin Type	Comments
Chattem Labs Mudd Super Cleansing Treatment	$	*, hydrated aluminum, magnesium silicate (clay), benzoin	oily	too drying for any but very oily skins; rinse-off clay mask, long-lasting
Barbara Walden Mint Masque	$$	*, lanolin, honey, mint	oily	rinse-off mask, softens skin but mint can irritate
Adrien Arpel Sea-Mud Pack	$$$	*, bentonite, SD alcohol 40	normal, oily	rinse-off clay; comes with applicator brush; leaves skin glowing; stains clothes
Orlane Ligne Active Masque Blue	$$$	*, bentonite, propylene glycol	oily, normal	rinse-off clay; very gentle for those with easily irritated skin
Elizabeth Arden Velva Cream Mask	$$	*, carrageen, glycerin	normal, sensitive, oily	clay rinse-off; very gentle
Revlon Moon Drops Honey Moisturizing Masque	$$	*, SD alcohol 40, polyvinyl, vinyl acetate copolymer	dry, normal	one of the few that work on dry skin; softens skin
Biotherm Masque Net	$$$	*, hydrolized animal protein, salicylic acid	normal	good for older skin

Product	Price	Ingredients	Skin type	Comments
Chanel Masque Lifting	$$$	*, polyvinyl	normal, dry	gentle, leaves a firming sensation (temporary)
Clarins Moisturizing Mask	$$	*, SD alcohol 40	dry, normal	creamy type
Lancôme Masque No. 10	$$$	*, fragancenth gum, algae extract, aloe extract, witch hazel	dry, sensitive	gel formulation
Orlane Ligne Integrale Masque Rose	$$$	*, petrolatum, bentonite	normal, on dry side	rinse-off clay; very gentle, has moistening effect on skin

Moisturizers

Product	Price	Ingredients	Skin type	Comments
Nutraderm	$	†, sorbitan stearate, mineral oil	normal, dry	lanolin-free, not greasy or sticky, forms light film, retarding moisture loss
Lubriderm	$	†, mineral oil, lanolin, lanolin alcohol	normal, dry	lanolin compounds may trouble acne
Neutrogena Moisture Lotion	$	†, petrolatum	normal, dry	water-based, light, nongreasy
Keri Lotion for Dry Skin Care	$	†, mineral oil, propylene glycol	normal, dry	very emollient
Vaseline Intensive Care	$	†, mineral oil	normal, dry	heavy, shiny finish

*In general, there are two types of masks: a mud/clay type or a vinyl type that peels; both usually have these ingredients suspended in a cream/lotion base.
†In general, moisturizers contain water, oil (petrolatum, mineral oil), waxes, emulsifying agents, preservatives.

Product	Price ($–$$$)	Ingredients of Note	Skin Type	Comments
Nivea Moisturizing Lotion	$	*, mineral oil, isopropyl myristate, lanolin oil	normal, dry	isopropyl myristate can aggravate acne
Noxell RainTree Lotion	$	*, oat flour	normal, dry	absorbs quickly, oat flour may fill in crinkles
Sea Breeze Moisture Lotion	$$	*, glycerin, aloe vera	normal, dry,	labeled "99% oil-free"
Youth Garde Moisturizer	$$	*, octyl palmitate, isopropylpalmitate PABA	normal, dry	can irritate skin of those sensitive to PABA; SPF 4
Almay Hypoallergenic Moisturizing Lotion	$$	*, glycerin	normal	quick absorption, nontacky finish
Wibi Lotion	$$	*, petrolatum	oily, acne-prone	light, ask at pharmacy counter
Cetaphil Cream	$$	*, cetyl alcohol	oily, acne-prone	ask at pharmacy counter
Allercreme Special Formula Lotion	$$	*, mineral oil	oily, acne-prone	lanolin-free, fragrance-free
Acquaderm (C & M Pharmacal)	$$	*, glycerin, salicyclic acid	oily, acne-prone	not tacky or sticky, oil-free
Colladerm (C&M)	$$	*, collagen, elastin, allantoin	oily, acne-prone	light, nongreasy finish, oil- and fat-free

Product	Price	Ingredients	Skin type	Notes
Dermalab Cream	$$	*	oily, acne-prone	doesn't exacerbate acne
Sea Breeze Moisture Lotion	$	*, isopropyl myristate	oily	oil-free formula
Revlon Moon Drops Moisture Film	$$	*, mineral oil, propylene glycol	oily	light lotion that absorbs quickly
Eucerin Lotion	$	*, mineral oil, isopropyl myristate, lanolin alcohol	dry, normal	unscented; can exacerbate acne
Complex 15 Moisturizing Face Cream Lotion	$$	*, glycerin, squalene	dry, normal, acne-prone	counters drying effects of acne medication
Dermik Labs Shephard's Lotion	$$	*, sesame oil, SD alcohol 40	oily, acne-prone	light formula, scented and unscented formulas
Biotherm Hydro-Normaliseur	$$$	*, glycerin	dry, mature, oily	oil-free, hydrating liquid
Lancôme Clarifiance	$$$	*, mineral oil	normal, dry	medium weight, quick absorption
Estée Lauder Non-Oily Skin Supplement	$$$	*, butylene glycol, soluable collagen extract	normal, oily	light, nonoily, matte finish
Doak Pharmaceutical Formula 405 Moisturizing Lotion	$$	*, sorbitol, stearic acid	normal	light, nongreasy, good under makeup

*In general, moisturizers contain water, oil (petrolatum, mineral oil), waxes, emulsifying agents, preservatives.

Product	Price ($–$$$)	Ingredients of Note	Skin Type	Comments
Pen-Kera (B.F.A. Ascher & Co.)	$$	*, cetyl palmitate, glycerin, mineral oil	dry	for chronic dry skin, fairly quick absorption
Oil of Olay Beauty Lotion	$	*, mineral oil, cholesterol	normal, dry, mature	glass bottle—watch for breaks
Nivea Moisturizing Lotion	$	*, glycerin, eucermite	normal	oil-in-water emulsion
Ponds Extra Rich Moisturizer Dry Skin Cream	$	*, petrolatum, mineral oil	dry	very emollient
Vaseline Dermatology Formula	$	*, petrolatum, mineral oil, dimethicone	dry	for very dry skin, shiny-smooth finish, nongreasy feel
Moisturel (Westwood)	$	*, petrolatum, glycerin	dry	paraben-free, fragrance-free, nongreasy
Lancôme Bienfait du Matin	$$$	*, hydrogenated polyisobutene, mineral oil	dry-normal	absorbs easily
Clinique Dramatically Different Moisturizing Lotion	$$$	*, mineral oil, sesame oil	dry-normal	absorbs slowly but velvety finish, basic product for problem-free skin, use under makeup
Clinique Skin Texture Lotion	$$$	*, soluable collagen extract, propylene glycol	oily	water-based, good under makeup

Product	Price	Ingredients	Skin Type	Characteristics
Clinque Very Emollient Cream	$$$	*, squalene, propylene glycol	dry	light, nontacky finish
Ultima II CHR Moisture Lotion Concentrate	$$$	*, propylene glycol, soluable collagen	dry, mature	dries to soft finish, rubs in quickly
Lancôme Hydrix Hydrating Cream	$$$	*, petrolalum, mineral oil, hydrated lanolin	dry, mature	heavy emollient formula, good staying power
Christian Dior Liquid Moisture Base	$$$	*, collagen, lanolin	normal, dry, mature	light, satiny feel
Revlon European Collagen Complex	$$	*, mineral oil, animal collagen complex	dry, mature	forms moisture-holding film
Flori Roberts Melanin Moisturizer	$$$	*	normal, dry	formulated for black/dark skin
Clarion Ultra Pure Moisturizer	$$	*	normal, dry	formulated for sensitive skin, dry finish, non-humectant formula
Shiseido B.H. 24 Day/Night Essence	$$$	*, biohyularonic acid	normal, dry	ampoules, A.M. and P.M.; good staying power
Chanel Emulsion No. 1 Equilibrium Supplement	$$$	*, acetylated lanolin, amniotic fluid	dry	not for acne-prone skin

*In general, moisturizers contain water, oil (petrolatum, mineral oil), waxes, emulsifying agents, preservatives.

Product	Price ($–$$$)	Ingredients of Note	Skin Type	Comments
Prescriptives Flight Cream	$$$	•, mineral oil, glycolipids, phospholipids	dry	good for frequent fliers or anyone in a very dry environment, very lubricating and emollient
Biotherm Sheer Energie Active	$$$	•, lanolin, benzophenone, methoxycinnamate	dry, normal	PABA-free sunscreen protection (SPF 4)
Frances Denny Multi-Layer Moisturizer	$$	•, mineral oil, glycerin	dry, very dry	contains sunscreen
Foundations				
Helena Rubinstein Liquid Silk Foundation	$$	†, mineral oil	dry	good coverage
Revlon Natural Wonder "Fresh All Day" Moisturizing Makeup	$	†, mineral oil	dry	light texture
Almay Protectives Lasting Finish Liquid Makeup	$	†, "cell energizing complex"	dry	good staying power
Max Factor Maxi Fresh Moisturizing Makeup	$	†, mineral oil	dry-mature	good coverage of crinkles, small lines without cakiness

Product	Price	Ingredients†	Skin type	Notes
Maybelline Mousse Makeup	$	†, water, isobutane	dry	very sheer coverage, mousse formula is fun, generally streakfree application; avoid eye area when spraying.
Allercreme Satin Finish Makeup	$	†, mineral oil	dry	fragrance-free, good coverage and finish
Almay Fresh Color Moisture Makeup	$	†, mineral oil	dry	fresh, dewy finish
Ultima II Actives Protective Face Color Mousse	$$	†, isobutane	dry-mature	SPF 6, sheer finish
Clarins Revitalizing Tinted Moisturizers	$$$	†, allantoin, cell extracts	dry-normal	4 tints, very sheer finish, not full coverage
Estée Lauder Fresh Air Makeup Base	$$$	†, propylene glycol	normal, oily	good coverage, matte finish, oil-free
Max Factor Creme Puff Makeup	$	†, talc, lanolin, beeswax, calcium carbonate	normal	light liquid
Almay Maximum Protection Cream-Powder Makeup	$	†, talc, PABA	normal	SPF 15

*In general, moisturizers contain water, oil (petrolatum, mineral oil), waxes, emulsifying agents, preservatives.
†In general, foundations consist of water and oil/wax with pigments (titanium dioxide, iron oxide) added. Magnesium aluminum silicate or talc indicates a matte finish.

Product	Price ($–$$$)	Ingredients of Note	Skin Type	Comments
Lancôme Bienfait de Matin Multi-protective Day Creme	$$	*, mineral oil, talc	normal, dry	light, tinted moisturizer; best for minimal coverage; spot application
Clinique Face Zone Sun Block	$$	*, PABA	normal, dry	tinted sunscreen; SPF 15
Biotherme Teint Tonic Protective Moisturizer	$$$	*, talc, kaolin	normal, dry	tinted moisturizer
Clinique Balanced Make Up Base	$$	*, mineral oil, propylene	dry	thick, creamy, labeled "hypoallergenic"
Chanel Teint Natural Liquid Make Up	$$$	*, talc, mineral oil, nylon	dry, normal	creamy, six shades, glowing finish
Shiseido Moisture Mist Foundation	$$$	*, talc, mineral oil	dry, normal	eight shades (looks darker on skin than in the bottle); light, creamy texture; matte finish
Ultima II ProCollagen Anti-Aging Firming Foundation	$$$	*, procollagen	dry, mature	creamy, moisturizing, medium heavy coverage
Estée Lauder Polished Performance Liquid Make Up	$$$	*, mineral oil, lanolin alcohol, PABA	dry, normal	water-based; fourteen shades; sunscreen; light sheer coverage and formulation

Product	Price	Ingredients	Skin type	Notes
Lancôme Dual Finish Cream/Powder Make Up	$$$	*, talc, mica, lanolin	all	oily, use it dry; others use it wet
Ultima II Beautiful Nutrient Make Up	$$$	*, propylene glycol, isoproyl myristate, quaternium 14, laureth 4	normal, oily	matte finish; not for acne-prone skin
Almay Fresh Look Oil-Free Makeup	$	*, water, glycerin, talc	oily, acne-prone	loose iron oxide powder in suspension—shake thoroughly before applying
Almay Smart Cover Makeup	$	*, glycerin, talc, kaolin	oily, acne-prone	light, can wear with medicated acne products
Helena Rubinstein Bio-Clear	$$	*, water, propylene glycol	oily, acne-prone	very light finish
Revlon Natural Wonder Oil Free Base	$	*, talc, isostearyl neopentanoate	oily	may exacerbate some cases of acne
Allercreme Matte Finish	$	*, talc	oily, acne-prone	matte finish
Maybelline Shine Free Oil Control Dual Powder Base	$	*, kaolin, titanium dioxide	oily	apply wet or dry for different effects
Cover Girl Oily Control Make Up	$	*, myristyl myristate, decyl oleate, clove oil, eucalyptus oil	oily	applies and wears well; finish is matte; good texture on skin

*In general, foundations consist of water and oil/wax with pigments (titanium dioxide, iron oxide) added. Magnesium aluminum silicate or talc indicates a matte finish.

Product	Price ($–$$$)	Ingredients of Note	Skin Type	Comments
Lancôme Macquicontrolle Oil-Free Liquid Make-Up	$$$	*, stearic acid, magnesium aluminum stearate, triethanolamine	oily	aromatic oils can irritate sensitive skin
Clinique Workout Makeup	$$$	*, cyclomethicone, propylene glycol, petrolatum	normal, mildly oily	great staying power
Janet Sartin Day Wear Astringent	$$$	*, SD alcohol 40, talc	oily, acne-prone	essentially a tinted astringent; good light coverage
Germaine Monteil Visage Clarité	$$$	*, cyclomethicone, glycerin	oily	matte finish medium texture and coverage
Ultima II Formula 2 Make Up	$$$	*, isopropyl palmitate	oily	medium texture
Elizabeth Arden Extra Control for Oily Skin	$$	*, SD alcohol 40	oily, acne-prone	oil-free; labeled "dermatologist, clinically and allergy tested"
Clinique Pore Minimizer Makeup	$$	*, SD alcohol 40, propylene glycol, talc, kaolin	oily to very oily	great for minimizing large pores, smooth finish
Prescriptives Oil Free Exact Color Makeup	$$	*, cyclomethicone, talc	oily, acne-prone	color mixed to your exact skin tone, good coverage without a heavy look or feel

Product	Price	Ingredients	Skin Type	Comments
Estée Lauder Oil Control Formula	$$	*, cyclomethicone, talc	oily	keeps "shiny nose" syndrome at bay very well; wears a long time
Chanel Oil Free Makeup	$$$	*, kaolin	oily, acne-prone	great texture, easy to apply, fine finish
Erno Lazlo Normalizing "Shake It" Foundation	$$$	*, SD alcohol 40, glycerin	oily, acne-prone	light but good coverage; may irritate those sensitive to lanolin; must invest in an initial membership before buying products
Clinique Stay-True Foundation	$$	*, cyclomethicone, kaolin	oily, acne-prone	nice matte finish, oil-free
Almay Moisturizing Foundation	$	*, mineral oil	sensitive	fragrance-free, preservative-free
Allercreme Matte, Velvet, and Satin Finish Makeup	$	*, titanium dioxide	sensitive oily (Matte Finish) normal (Velvet Finish) dry (Satin Finish)	fragrance-free, labeled "hypoallergenic," light texture
Noxell Clarion Ultra Pure Foundation	$$	*, propylene glycol	sensitive	fragrance-free, sheer finish
Clinique Balanced Makeup Base	$$	*, mineral oil, propylene glycol	sensitive	very light texture

*In general, foundations consist of water and oil/wax with pigments (titanium dioxide, iron oxide) added. Magnesium aluminum silicate or talc indicates a matte finish.

Product	Price ($–$$$)	Ingredients of Note	Skin Type	Comments
Estée Lauder Soft Finish Compact Makeup	$$	*, phenyltrimethicone, talc	sensitive	good for slightly dry skin, matte finish, good for touch-ups, spot coverage

Powders

Product	Price ($–$$$)	Ingredients of Note	Skin Type	Comments
Coty Correctives Powder	$	†, talc, zinc oxide, witch hazel extract	oily, acne-prone	great coverage, blots oil well
Maybelline Shine Free Oil Control Dual Base Powder	$	†, mineral oil, talc	normal, oily	tinted powder; substantial enough to be used alone, without foundation
Max Factor Ultralucent Ultra Sheer Face Powder	$	†, talc	oily, normal	translucent
Cover Girl Translucent Blotting Powder	$	†, oat flour, zinc stearate, clove/eucalptus oil, mineral oil	mildly oily, normal	aromatic oils can irritate sensitive skin
Revlon Skin Balancing Powder	$$	†, talc, mineral oil	dry	matte finish, soft texture
Almay Translucent Finish Face Power	$	†, talc, magnesium stearate	normal	ultralight, fine sheer finish
Almay Shine Free Blotting Powder	$	†, talc, hydrated silica, kaolin	oily	good absorption properties; fragrance-free

Product	Price	Ingredients	Skin Type	Comments
Allercreme Translucent Loose Face Powder	$	†, talc, magnesium stearale, iron oxides	normal, sensitive	natural, sheer finish
Chanel Poudre Douce	$$$	†, talc, silk powder, polyethylene	normal, mildly oily	extremely velvety; good natural coverage; silk powder a possible irritant
Lancôme Boite A Poudre	$$$	†, magnesium carbonate, acacia	normal, mildly oily	good finish, unique dispenser keeps you from pouring out too much
Alexandra de Markoff Finishing Powder	$$$	†, talc, rice starch, magnesium carbonate	normal, dry	good coverage and finish
Shiseido Green Moisture Mist Compact Foundation	$$$	†, talc, mineral oil	normal, oily	ultrafine texture and finish
Lancôme Macquifinish Pressed Powder Translucent Matte	$$$	†, talc	normal, oily	mirrored compact; very light; matte finish with nice glow to it

*In general, foundations consist of water and oil/wax with pigments (titanium dioxide, iron oxide) added. Magnesium aluminum silicate or talc indicates a matte finish.
†In general, powders consist of a base (talc, magnesium, aluminum silicate) with pigment. Zinc stearate aids the adherence of powder to skin.

INDEX

References to illustrations are in boldface

ABOUT THE AUTHORS

THOMAS GOODMAN, M.D., began a career in research and teaching, that evolved into a private practice. He has published many articles in scientific journals, and he holds a faculty appointment at the University of Tennessee Center for the Health Sciences. He is a consultant in dermatology to several hospitals, a fellow of the American Academy of Dermatology, and a member of several other medical societies.

Now, in addition to his busy private practice, he is devoting more time to his interests in writing and research. Dr. Goodman is involved in developing new drugs for the treatment of acne and other skin diseases and in developing new skin-care products.

Dr. Goodman lives and works in Memphis, Tennessee.

STEPHANIE YOUNG graduated from Stanford University in 1978 with a B.A. in English, with distinction. She was on staff at *Mademoiselle* magazine for two years and was a beauty and health writer at *Glamour* magazine for five years. She is a contributor to *American Health* magazine and is currently a free-lance writer specializing in the health and beauty field. She lives in New York City.